School-Based Mental Health Services

SCHOOL PSYCHOLOGY
BOOK SERIES

School-Based Mental Health Services

Creating Comprehensive and Culturally Specific Programs

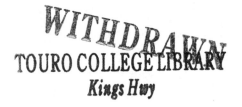

Bonnie Kaul Nastasi, Rachel Bernstein Moore, and Kristen M. Varjas

American Psychological Association
Washington, DC

KH

Published by
American Psychological Association
750 First Street, NE
Washington, DC 20002
www.apa.org

To order
APA Order Department
P.O. Box 92984
Washington, DC 20090-2984
Tel: (800) 374-2721
Direct: (202) 336-5510
Fax: (202) 336-5502
TDD/TTY: (202) 336-6123
Online: www.apa.org/books/
E-mail: order@apa.org

In the U.K., Europe, Africa, and the Middle East, copies may be ordered from
American Psychological Association
3 Henrietta Street
Covent Garden, London
WC2E 8LU England

Typeset in Goudy by World Composition Services, Inc., Sterling, VA

Printer: Sheridan Books, Ann Arbor, MI
Cover Designer: NiDesign, Baltimore, MD
Technical/Production Editor: Dan Brachtesende

Library of Congress Cataloging-in-Publication Data

Nastasi, Bonnie K.
　　School-based mental health services : creating comprehensive and culturally specific programs / Bonnie K. Nastasi, Rachel B. Moore, Kristen M. Varjas.—1st ed.
　　　　p. cm.—(Applying psychology to the schools)
　　Includes bibliographical references and indexes.
　　ISBN 1-59147-018-8
　　1. Child mental health services—United States. 2. School children—Mental health services—United States. 3. Teenagers—Mental health services—United States. 4. Psychiatry, Transcultural—United States. I. Moore, Rachel B. II. Varjas, Kristen M. III. Title. IV. Series.

RJ501.A2N28　2003
362.2′083′0973—dc22　　　　　　　　　　　　　　　　　　　　　　　　2003013782

British Library Cataloguing-in-Publication Data
A CIP record is available from the British Library.

Printed in the United States of America
First Edition

10/25/04

We dedicate this book to children and adolescents and their caregivers worldwide, that they might have available to them the personal and social–cultural resources necessary for promoting mental health and psychological well-being for themselves and others.

CONTENTS

FIGURES, TABLES, AND EXHIBITS

FIGURES

TABLES

EXHIBITS

PREFACE

The mental health needs of children and adolescents within the United States and worldwide have received increasing attention in recent years. As we discuss in chapter 1, it is estimated that approximately one fifth of America's children and adolescents have diagnosable disorders that require mental health treatment. Internationally, it is expected that mental illness will become one of the five most common causes of childhood disability, morbidity, or mortality within the next 20 years. These figures do not include those children and adolescents who are at risk for, or currently experiencing, mental health problems that do not warrant diagnosis but nevertheless affect everyday functioning and well-being or those who experience social morbidities, such as drug abuse, sexual risk, child abuse, and family and community violence, which increase the risk for mental health problems.

Despite the prevalence of mental health difficulties and social morbidities, many children and adolescents do not receive treatment in the health sector because of factors such as lack of health insurance, poverty, stigma, and lack of culturally appropriate services. Schools provide an alternative site for the provision of comprehensive mental health services, including mental health promotion, risk reduction, early intervention, and treatment, which can benefit all students. In addition, schools can play a critical role in the coordination of efforts among various stakeholders, including parents, community organizations, hospitals, community mental health facilities, and other social service agencies. Research supports the effectiveness of comprehensive and coordinated mental health service delivery. Realization of such efforts, however, is hindered by the shortage of models for translating research to practice and for addressing the cultural diversity that characterizes the U.S. population. The combination of these factors provided the impetus for development and application of the participatory culture-specific intervention model (PCSIM), which is described in this book. We anticipate that this work will make a critical contribution to the literature on school-based mental health service delivery and facilitate the involvement of key stakeholders in the development and implementation of culturally specific mental health programming for all students.

This book is designed for practitioners, researchers, and graduate students who are interested in meeting the mental health needs of children and adolescents in the 21st century through comprehensive school-based programming. We present a model, the PCSIM, to guide the development, implementation, and evaluation of school-based mental health services. The PCSIM represents an integration of research and intervention that is consistent with current concepts of science-based psychological practice, incorporates characteristics of effective comprehensive programming, and provides guidelines for developing culturally specific services. The text addresses the multiple roles of program partners (e.g., researchers, evaluators, interventionists, support personnel), with particular attention to psychologists or other mental health professionals who will assume leadership in the application of PCSIM. We provide background information on mental health needs of children and adolescents and research on the effectiveness of comprehensive programming. Most of the text is devoted to the description of PCSIM, its key components, and delineation of the procedures for the application of PCSIM in school settings. The inclusion of step-by-step procedures, practical tools, and examples from real-life application is expected to facilitate the implementation of PCSIM. Although the specific focus of the book is creating school-based mental health services, the PCSIM has broader application to developing community-based health and mental health services. Furthermore, recognizing the interdisciplinary nature of comprehensive programming, we advocate the involvement of professionals from multiple fields such as psychology, medicine, education, social work, public health, anthropology, and sociology. Because of the scope of PCSIM and comprehensive mental health programming, professionals from disciplines within mental health, health, education, and social services are likely to find this book useful.

ACKNOWLEDGMENTS

We extend our gratitude to the children, adolescents, and adults who have contributed to our research and professional practice and whose experiences have advanced our knowledge about mental health and have provided the illustrations in this text. We extend special thanks to Dr. Asoka Jayasena, University of Peradeniya, Sri Lanka, her faculty colleagues and graduate students, and the students and staff of the Central Province schools in Sri Lanka. Our work in Sri Lanka provided the inspiration and foundation for the development of the participatory culture-specific intervention model. We also thank the numerous graduate students at the University at Albany, State University of New York and Georgia State University in Atlanta who contributed to the background work reflected in this text. Our gratitude also is extended to Sandra Christenson and Sue Sheridan, series editors; Kristine Enderle, development editor, and Dan Brachtesende, production editor at the American Psychological Association; and Stephen Leff, Cherie Tyler Balkcom, and Suzanne Margiano, for their critiques and suggestions during the development of this volume.

School-Based
Mental Health Services

1

MEETING THE MENTAL HEALTH NEEDS OF CHILDREN AND ADOLESCENTS

Promoting mental health for all Americans will require scientific know-how but, even more importantly, a societal resolve that we will make the needed investment. The investment does not call for massive budgets; rather, it calls for the willingness of each of us to educate ourselves and others about mental health and mental illness, and thus to confront the attitudes, fear, and misunderstanding that remain as barriers before us. (U.S. Surgeon General David Satcher; U.S. Department of Health and Human Services [USDHHS], 1999, p. vi)

As professionals working in schools, psychologists can play an important role in confronting attitudes, fears, and misunderstandings that prohibit adequate attention to mental health in society. Furthermore, school psychologists are in a unique position to advocate for development, implementation, and evaluation of school-based mental health promotion, intervention, and treatment programs and to ensure that science-based strategies are used.

FOCUS OF THE BOOK

Described herein is a participatory process for creating or facilitating the development of acceptable, socially valid, effective, and sustainable programs. The *participatory culture-specific intervention model* (PCSIM) is a general model for developing interventions that can be applied to a range of settings, populations, and target problems. In this text, the model is described and illustrated with reference to providing comprehensive school-based mental health services. Although the text is directed primarily to psychologists working in schools, the intended audience includes the full range of school professionals who have responsibility for development and evaluation of mental health services. The creation and implementation of comprehensive mental health services is not a task that can be accomplished by one individual (e.g., a school psychologist working alone). Indeed, the participatory nature of the process necessitates the collaboration of professionals and nonprofessionals who have vested interests and resources relevant to students' well-being. In addition, the scope of the work requires the expertise, time, and energy of multiple individuals. Furthermore, the development of sustainable programs entails long-term commitment from key stakeholders and agencies.

The purpose of this text is to provide a guide for psychologists and other mental health professionals who are interested in developing or are currently engaged in providing comprehensive school-based mental health services. Although the task of providing comprehensive services to children and adolescents is daunting, it is not impossible. To facilitate effective planning and implementation, we provide a step-by-step process that begins with system entry and culminates in program continuation–extension. The focus is development of comprehensive, systemwide programs; however, this does not preclude professionals from applying the strategies and principles to work on a smaller scale, and we provide illustrations for both full-scale programming and more focused application.

This first chapter addresses three key questions: Why are school-based mental health services necessary? What constitutes comprehensive mental health services in schools? How can psychologists contribute to school-based mental health promotion and intervention efforts? Before addressing these questions, we examine current definitions of mental health, mental health problems, and mental illness as proposed by the U.S. Surgeon General (USDHHS, 1999).

MENTAL HEALTH AS PUBLIC HEALTH

In contrast to past dichotomies of mental health and illness, current thinking is characterized by a health–illness continuum (USDHHS, 1999). Mental health, mental health problems, and mental illness or disorders are viewed as points along a continuum. For our purposes, we adopt the definitions of mental health, mental illness, and mental health problems set forth by the U.S. Surgeon General (USDHHS, 1999; see Exhibit 1.1). Mental health, like health, is "rooted in a population-based public health model" (USDHHS, 1999, p. 7). In contrast to the traditional medical model, which is focused on diagnosis, treatment, and etiology, the contemporary public health model advocated by the USDHHS is focused more broadly on surveillance of mental health within the population at large, mental health promotion and illness prevention, person–environment links,

Mental health is a state of successful performance of mental function, resulting in productive activities, fulfilling relationships with other people, and the ability to adapt to change and to cope with adversity. Mental health is indispensable to personal well-being, family and interpersonal relationships, and contribution to community or society. It is easy to overlook the value of mental health until problems surface. Yet from early childhood until death, mental health is the springboard of thinking and communication skills, learning, emotional growth, resilience, and self-esteem. These are the ingredients of each individual's successful contribution to community and society. Americans are inundated with messages about success—in school, in a profession, in parenting, in relationships—without appreciating that successful performance rests on a foundation of mental health. (USDHHS, 1999, p. 4)

Mental illness is the term that refers collectively to all diagnosable mental disorders. Mental disorders are health conditions that are characterized by alterations in thinking, mood, or behavior (or some combination thereof) associated with distress and/or impaired functioning. . . . Alterations in thinking, mood, or behavior contribute to a host of problems—patient distress, impaired functioning, or heightened risk of death, pain, disability, or loss of freedom (*DSM–IV,* 1994 [American Psychiatric Association, 1994]). (USDHHS, 1999, p. 5)

Mental health problems (is the term used) for signs and symptoms of insufficient intensity or duration to meet the criteria for any mental disorder. Almost everyone has experienced mental health problems in which the distress one feels matches some of the signs and symptoms of mental disorders. Mental health problems may warrant active efforts in health promotion, prevention, and treatment. . . . (In some cases) early intervention is needed to address a mental health problem before it becomes a potentially life-threatening disorder. (USDHHS, 1999, p. 5)

access to services, and evaluation of services. A public health perspective thus implies (a) comprehensive service provision, characterized by a continuum of services (from prevention to treatment); (b) an ecological model that takes into account social, cultural, and physical environmental factors; (c) provision of services that are easily accessed by the general population, for example, through public facilities such as schools; (d) a science-based approach to practice that includes ongoing evaluation; and (e) methods for surveillance of mental health needs. Given the scope of a public health model, collaboration within and across disciplinary lines is necessary. The model for school-based mental health presented in this book embodies all of these dimensions.

THE NEED FOR MENTAL HEALTH SERVICES IN SCHOOLS

In 1990, it was estimated that 15% to 22% of U.S. children and adolescents had mental health problems that were serious enough to warrant diagnosis and treatment (National Advisory Mental Health Council, 1990; National Institute of Mental Health [NIMH], 1990; Zill & Schoenborn, 1990). The 1999 USDHHS report by the U.S. Surgeon General confirms the continued need for mental health services for children and adolescents. Furthermore, more recent efforts through the President's New Freedom Commission on Mental Health (Office of the Press Secretary, 2002) reflect sustained interest in the mental health needs of American children.

PSYCHIATRIC DISORDERS

According to the U.S. Surgeon General (USDHHS, 1999), approximately 20% of U.S. children and adolescents experience symptoms of diagnosable mental disorders (i.e., psychiatric disorders, according to the 4th ed. of the *Diagnostic and Statistical Manual of Mental Disorders* [DSM–IV]; American Psychiatric Association, 1994) over a one-year period, although only 5% are considered to be experiencing extreme functional impairment. The incidence over the course of a year is comparable for adults (20%); however, 15% of adults with mental disorders also have a co-occurring substance abuse disorder. Adolescents who experience mental health problems or other health problems related to social and behavioral factors (i.e., social morbidities such as alcohol or drug abuse, pregnancy, physical injury, or fear of violence) are "less likely to learn, irrespective of efforts to improve educational methods, standards, or organizations" (Kolbe, Collins, & Cortese, 1997, p. 256). Furthermore, the mental health problems of children and adolescents have potentially far-reaching effects, as suggested by the following statement from the NIMH (1999):

> Recent evidence compiled by the World Health Organization indicates that by the year 2020, childhood neuropsychiatric disorders will rise proportionately by over 50 percent, internationally, to become one of the five most common causes of morbidity, mortality, and disability among children. (para. 1)

Epidemiological research in the past decade confirms the U.S. Surgeon General's call for increased attention to mental health as a national and global priority. According to Doll (1996), diagnosable psychiatric disorders occur in approximately 180 to 200 per thousand school-age children, with the most prevalent being anxiety and behavior disorders, and for secondary-level students, depression and suicidal behavior. The National Association of School Psychologists (NASP, 1997) estimated that 20% of school-age children have significant mental health problems and that 50% of adolescents are at moderate to high risk for such problems. The NIMH (1999) reported that 10% of children and adolescents in the United States have mental health problems that are severe enough to impair functioning. In particular, the NIMH estimates that as many as 3% of children and 8% of adolescents in the United States experience depression; as many as 13% of the school-age population have an anxiety disorder over a one-year period; an estimated 3% to 5% of school-age children are affected by attention deficit hyperactivity disorders (ADHDs); and 1% of the adolescent population (ages 14–18) meet the criteria for manic-depressive illness or its milder form, cyclothymia, during their lifetime. Furthermore, schizophrenia, which typically emerges in late adolescence or early adulthood, affects approximately 1% of the population.

SOCIAL MORBIDITIES

In addition to psychiatric disorders, school-age youths also experience a range of social morbidities and health risks. Social morbidities are health problems resulting from behavioral, social, and environmental factors related to lifestyle (DiClemente, Hansen, & Ponton, 1996), such as suicide, substance (tobacco, alcohol, and other drugs) abuse and its related unintentional injuries (e.g., motor vehicle injuries), sexual risks (e.g., pregnancy), sexually transmitted diseases (STDs, including HIV/AIDS), physical and sexual abuse, homelessness, school dropout or refusal, eating disorders, and community and domestic violence and related homicide and victimization. The inclusion of social morbidities within the category of mental health concerns increases the scope of the problem. Kolbe et al. (1997) suggested that the most serious and expensive health and social problems in the United States are caused primarily by behavioral patterns established prior to adulthood. In particular, they identified six behavioral categories as causal factors in major health problems: (a) those related to intentional or unintentional injury, (b) drug and alcohol abuse, (c) sexual behaviors that cause STDs or unintended pregnancy, (d) inadequate exercise, (e) dietary patterns that cause disease, and (f) tobacco use. Similarly, the NIMH (1990) suggested that child and adolescent psychiatric disorders arise from the complex interaction of biological, psychological, and social ("biopsychosocial") factors.

According to the Centers for Disease Control and Prevention (CDC, 2002b) report of the 2001 Youth Risk Behavior Surveillance System (YRBSS) data (for the period of February–December, 2001), social morbidities accounted for the majority of deaths (71%) for children and youth ages 10 to 24: motor vehicle crashes, 31%; other unintentional injuries, 12%; homicides, 15%; and suicides, 12%. Preliminary national statistics regarding deaths for 1999 (Kochanek, Smith, & Anderson, 1999) revealed the following figures: ages 5 to 14, 1.1 per 100,000 died by homicide, 0.6 by suicide, and 7.8 by unintentional injuries (4.8 related to motor vehicle accidents);

ages 15 to 24, 13.2 per 100,000 died by homicide, 10.3 by suicide, and 36 by unintentional injuries (26.8 related to motor vehicle accidents).

Suicide

Suicide has been identified as the third leading cause of death for adolescents and young adults (ages 15–24) and the fourth leading cause of death for children ages 5 to 14 years (Malley, Kush, & Bogo, 1994; NIMH, 1999; Sells & Blum, 1996). It is estimated that a child commits suicide every 90 minutes; this figure includes a disproportionate number of special education students (NASP, 1997). Furthermore, the suicide rate for adolescents and young adults has increased by 200% to 300% over the 30-year period from the 1960s to 1990s (Malley et al., 1994; NIMH, 1999).

Deaths by suicide do not accurately estimate the number of attempts, however, as less than 1 in 50 attempts results in death (Sells & Blum, 1996). In response to the national YRBSS surveys (administered February to December, 2001; Grades 9 through 12, $N = 13,601$; CDC, 2002b), 8.8% of high school students (female students, 11.2%; male students, 6.2%) reported attempting suicide at least one time during the preceding 12 months, and 2.6% (female students, 3.1%; male students, 2.1%) reported making a suicide attempt (during the same period) resulting in injury, overdose, or poisoning that required medical treatment. In addition, 14.8% (female students, 17.7%; male students, 11.8%) reported serious suicide ideation (i.e., had made a specific plan), 19% (female students, 23.6%; male students, 14.2%) seriously considered attempting suicide, and 28.3% (female students, 34.5%; male students, 21.6%) reported feeling sad or hopeless enough to discontinue some usual activities (CDC, 2002b). Furthermore, depression in children and adolescents has been linked to increased risk of suicide; and among adolescent boys, this risk is increased when depression co-occurs with conduct disorder and alcohol or substance abuse (NIMH, 2000).

Violence

Researchers, educators, mental health practitioners, and community members have become increasingly concerned about the impact of school and community violence on youths. More than 4,000 children and teens were killed by gunfire in 1997 (Children's Defense Fund, 2000); every day 10 to 15 children are killed by firearms (Children's Defense Fund, 1999; NASP, 1997). Homicide has been identified as the second leading cause of death for adolescents and young adults (ages 15–24) in the United States, with a rate of 20.3 per 100,000 (R. N. Anderson, Kochanek, & Murphy, 1997), and the third leading cause of death among children ages 5 to 14 (Children's Defense Fund, 1999). In 1999, the rate of serious violent crime (i.e., aggravated assault, rape, and robbery) against youths ages 12 to 17 was 20 per 1,000, a rate twice that for adults (Federal Interagency Forum on Child and Family Statistics, 2001). In a 1999 study of 94 inner-city adolescents, 93% of the respondents reported that they had been exposed to at least one community violent event (Mazza & Reynolds, 1999).

Seven percent of high school students responding to the YRBSS survey between February and December 2001 indicated they missed one or more days of school (over the preceding month) because of feeling unsafe, 9% were threatened or injured with a weapon at school (during the preceding year), and 13% engaged in a physical fight on school property (during the preceding year; CDC, 2002b). Furthermore, 10% of the students reported being victims of dating violence (i.e., being hit, slapped, or physically hurt on purpose by boyfriend–girlfriend; female students, 10%; male students, 9%), and 8% reported forced sexual intercourse (i.e., being forced to have sexual intercourse when they did not want to). Reported incidence of forced sexual intercourse against female students (11%) was more than twice that against male students (5%).

In addition to school and community violence, youths are subjected to domestic violence such as physical or sexual abuse. The Children's Defense Fund (2000) reported that 3 million children were suspected victims of child abuse or neglect during 1997. More than 8,000 children are reported to be abused or neglected every day, and one in four girls and one in seven boys are sexually abused before the age of 18 (NASP, 1997). It has been estimated that 4% to 5% of children are victims of abuse or neglect annually in the United States (USDHHS, 1993).

Epidemiological research also documents the involvement of youths as perpetrators of violent crime. The rate of serious violent crimes committed by juvenile offenders (ages 12–17) in 1999 was 26 per 1,000 (Federal Interagency Forum on Child and Family Statistics, 2001). Nearly half (47%) of these crimes involved more than one juvenile offender; therefore, the number of juvenile offenders is actually higher (exact number undetermined). According to self-reports of violence (collected during February–December, 2001; CDC, 2002b), 33% of high school students (female students, 24%; male students, 43%) participated in one or more physical fights during the preceding 12 months, and 4% required medical treatment for injuries sustained in physical fights.

Increase in lethality of violent crimes committed by youthful offenders has been attributed to increase in handgun use (Sells & Blum, 1996). In the nationwide 2001 study of 13,601 high school students (CDC, 2002b), 17% (female students, 6%; male students, 29%) reported carrying a weapon (e.g., knife, gun, club) in the past month, 6% (female students, 1%; male students, 10%) reported carrying a gun, and 6% (female students, 3%; male students, 10%) reported carrying a weapon on school property. In another study of 750 inner-city high school youths (Sheley & Wright, 1995), 80% reported they had carried a weapon to school, 66% knew someone who had carried a weapon to school, and 65% indicated they could get a gun with little or no difficulty.

According to official records (e.g., arrest records), the unprecedented increase in juvenile violence from 1983 to 1993 was followed by a decline (USDHHS, 2001b). Confidential self-reports, however, suggest that the proportion of youths committing serious, and possibly lethal, acts of violence has remained at the 1993 peak. These figures, coupled with much publicized and tragic school shootings (e.g., Columbine High School, Colorado, April 1999), have prompted health and mental health officials to designate youth violence as a public health concern and to call for research and service provision related to violence prevention. Evidence of long-term effects of exposure to violence reinforces the need for such efforts.

The relationship between exposure to violence and mental health problems among children and adolescents is well documented (Berton & Stabb, 1996; Mazza & Overstreet, 2000; Osofsky, 1995). The effects of exposure to violence are not specific to a single domain of functioning (Berton & Stabb, 1996; Cicchetti & Lynch, 1993; DuRant, Cadenhead, Pendergrast, Slavens, & Linder, 1994; Fletcher, 1996; Mazza & Overstreet, 2000; Mazza & Reynolds, 1999; Osofsky, 1995; Schwab-Stone et al., 1995). Instead, violence exposure has both direct and indirect relationships to a range of mental health difficulties, problematic behaviors, and academic difficulties. Furthermore, exposure to violence has been identified as the strongest predictor of violence among adolescents (DuRant et al., 1994).

Peer victimization has received ever-increasing attention in the aftermath of school shootings that occurred in the United States during the 1990s. In particular, the association between prior victimization (feeling bullied, injured, or persecuted by others) of the perpetrator and targeted school violence (e.g., shooting of other students and teachers) has resulted in calls for efforts to reduce bullying in schools (Vossekuil, Fein, Reddy, Borum, & Modzeleski, 2002). Recent research has further documented the association among victimization, perpetration of violence, and mental health problems. For example, peer victimization has been associated with symptoms of anxiety and depression (Bond, Carlin, Thomas, Rubin, & Patton, 2001) and posttraumatic stress disorder (PTSD; Mynard, Joseph, & Alexander, 2000). Both victimization and bullying have been associated with anxiety, depression, eating disorders, and psychosomatic symptoms (Kaltiala-Heino, Rimpela, Rantanen, & Rimpela, 2000). Some research, however, suggests that victims of violence are more likely to experience internalizing problems, whereas perpetrators (i.e., bullies) are more likely to exhibit externalizing problems (Sourander, Helstela, Helenius, & Piha, 2000). In one study, intentions to use violence among adolescents were associated with prior exposure to violence, victimization by violence, substance use, depression, and interest in joining a gang (Barkin, Kreiter, & DuRant, 2001). Other research supports the association between substance abuse (e.g., excessive drinking) and bullying behavior among high school students (Kaltiala-Heino et al., 2000). Perhaps most important, both bullying and victimization have been identified as persistent behaviors, with victimization being the more persistent (Sourander et al., 2000). This finding, coupled with greater prevalence of bullying and victimization in elementary school (age 8) than in high school (age 16; Sourander et al., 2000), underscores the need for prevention and early intervention.

The far-reaching impact of exposure to violence is likely the result of PTSD symptomatology that leads to other problems (Mazza & Reynolds, 1999). Alternatively, exposure to community violence may result in disturbances within the family environment, which then alter the role of traditional compensatory factors and negatively influence child and adolescent functioning (e.g., in academic domain; Cicchetti & Lynch, 1993). PTSD diagnosis as well as exposure to violence and other psychological or social stressors (e.g., poverty, family disruption) have been associated with high rates of generalized anxiety, dissociative responses, depression and suicidal ideation, developmental and school or academic difficulties (e.g., retention, grades, achievement scores), and aggressive–violent and antisocial behavior (Berton & Stabb, 1996; Cicchetti & Lynch, 1993; DuRant et al., 1994; Fletcher, 1996; Garrison, Roy, & Azar, 1999; Mazza & Overstreet, 2000; Mazza & Reynolds, 1999; Osofsky, 1995; Schwab-Stone et al., 1995). An estimated 30% of preschoolers and 12% of elementary school children exposed to traumatic events engage in antisocial behavior (Fletcher, 1996).

Research on the risk factors associated with PTSD highlights the complexity of social morbidities (Friedman & Marsella, 1996). For example, poverty and parental divorce have been associated with increased vulnerability to PTSD. The degree of exposure to trauma (e.g., through repeated victimization) has been identified as the best predictor of PTSD. Furthermore, social–cultural factors such as family stability, community support, low rates of community drug use, and environmental safety have been associated with low risk for PTSD.

Drugs

Drug use and abuse by children and adolescents are of increasing professional and public concern. Researchers have suggested that alcohol is the most commonly used and abused drug among youths and that its use increases during adolescence (CDC, 2000b; Federal Interagency Forum on

TABLE 1.1
Lifetime and Current Drug Use by High School Students, 2001[a]

Drug	Lifetime[b]	Current[b]
Alcohol	78.2	47.1
All tobacco[c]	—	33.9
Cigarettes	63.9	28.5
Marijuana	42.4	23.9
Inhalants[d]	14.7	4.7
Cocaine	9.4	4.2
Heroin	3.1	—
Methamphetamine[e]	9.8	—
Steroids[f]	5.0	—
Injecting illegal drugs	2.3	—

Note. Figures represent percentage of students reporting use. Dashes = data not reported.
[a]On the basis of the 2001 nationwide Youth Risk Behavior Surveillance System survey of 13,601 high school students, Grades 9 to 12, administered from February to December; reported by the Centers for Disease Control and Prevention (2002b). [b]Lifetime use = at least once during their lifetime. Current use = one or more time during the preceding 30 days. [c]Cigarettes, smokeless tobacco, and cigars. [d]Breathe contents of aerosol cans, or inhale paints or spray to get high. [e]Addictive stimulant drug. [f]Illegal use, that is, without doctor's prescription.

Child and Family Statistics, 2001; Johnston, O'Malley, & Bachman, 2001a, 2001b; Sells & Blum, 1996). Statistics from the year 2000 indicated alcohol use by 50% of 12th graders in the preceding 30 days, 41% of 10th graders, and 22% of 8th graders (Johnston et al., 2001a, 2001b). Rates of heavy drinking (i.e., at least five drinks in a row at least once in the previous 2 weeks) among high school students reflect similar increases with age, with 30% of 12th graders, 26% of 10th graders, and 14% of 8th graders reporting heavy drinking in the 2000 Monitoring the Future Study (Johnston et al., 2001a, 2001b).

Table 1.1 includes drug use data from the YRBSS survey administered to 13,601 high school students, Grades 9 to 12, between February and December 2001 (CDC, 2002b). As the figures indicate, alcohol is the most commonly used drug, followed by tobacco and marijuana. The majority (78%) of high school students reported lifetime alcohol use (at least one alcoholic drink during their lifetime; Table 1.1), 47% reported current alcohol use (one or more drinks over the preceding 30 days; Table 1.1), and 30% reported episodic heaving drinking (five or more drinks on at least one occasion during the preceding 30 days). Almost one third (29%) of the respondents reported having consumed alcohol before the age of 13. In addition, the majority (64%) of students had tried cigarettes (22% before the age of 13), and close to half (42%; 10% before age 13) had smoked marijuana. Fewer adolescents reported using heroine, methamphetamine, steroids, and injecting drugs (see Table 1.1).

In recent years, increasing use of so-called "club drugs," such as MDMA (3-4-methylenedioxymethamphetamine, a synthetic drug with amphetaminelike and hallucinogenic properties, commonly known as Ecstasy), has incited concern among professionals and lay public. In 2000, 7.3% of 10th graders and 11% of 12th graders reported lifetime use of Ecstasy (Johnston et al., 2001a). Comparable figures for previous years are 5.7% and 6.9% in 1997, 5.1% and 5.8% in 1998, and 6.0% and 8.0% in 1999, for 10th and 12th graders, respectively (Johnston et al., 2001b). In response to the increasing popularity of club drugs among youths, researchers and interventionists have begun to include them in drug prevention programs (e.g., Nastasi et al., 2001).

Availability of drugs in and around schools, despite efforts to establish drug-free zones, is another issue of increasing concern. Data from the 2001 (February–December) YRBSS survey suggest that youths not only use drugs on school grounds but also can acquire illegal drugs at school (CDC, 2002b). Nationwide, 10% of high school students indicated they had smoked cigarettes on school property within the preceding 30 days, 5% had used smokeless tobacco, 4.9% had used alcohol, and 5.4% had used marijuana (during the preceding 30 days). During the preceding 12 months, 28.5% of the respondents had been given, offered, or sold an illegal drug on the school grounds.

In a study by the Institute for Community Research (J. J. Schensul, 2001), 70% of self-identified drug-using urban youths (ages 16 to 25) reported that it was easy or very easy to get alcohol in or around school; 91% indicated it was easy or very easy to get marijuana; 39%, heroin; and 54%, cocaine or crack. Seventy-three percent of this sample of 401 youths reported lifetime involvement, and 31% reported current involvement in drug-related activities.

Of primary concern with regard to drug use, particularly alcohol and tobacco, are the immediate and long-term health risks such as disease, disability, and death (Federal Interagency Forum on Child and Family Statistics, 2001). One particular concern related to adolescent (and adult) alcohol use is the risk associated with driving after drinking (CDC, 2002b). Approximately one third (30.7%) of high school students reported having ridden (during the preceding 30 days) with a driver who had been drinking; and 13% reported driving (during the preceding 30 days) after drinking alcohol (CDC, 2002b).

Other researchers have linked alcohol use to motor vehicle accidents. Using statistics from the U.S. Department of Transportation, Sells and Blum (1996) suggested that youths ages 16 to 20 (compared with any other age group) who were involved in fatal crashes were more likely to have been alcohol impaired.

Sexual Activity

Research confirms the need for concern about sexual risks among youths in the United States. The majority of youths are sexually active by age 18, and as many as 10% initiate sexual intercourse before the age of 13 (CDC, 2000b, 2002b; Sells & Blum, 1996). Almost half (45.6% total; 42.9% of female students, 49% of male students) of the high school students (Grades 9–12) responding to the 2001 YRBSS survey reported that they had had sexual intercourse during their lifetime (CDC, 2002b). By Grade 9, 29.1% of female students and 34.4% of male students had had sexual intercourse; by Grade 12, percentages increased to 60.1% for female students and 61% for male students. Fourteen percent of all students (female students, 11%; male students, 17%) reported having had sexual intercourse with multiple partners (four or more) during their lifetime. Initiation into sexual intercourse before the age of 13 was reported more frequently by male students (9.3%) than female students (4%); the overall level was 6.6%. One third (33.4%) of all students reported that they were currently sexually active (i.e., had sexual intercourse during the preceding 3 months).

Among sexually active respondents, the majority (58%; female students, 51%; male students, 65%) reported condom use by themselves or their partners during their last sexual intercourse (CDC, 2002b). Fewer than 20% (18.2%; female students, 21%; male students, 15%) reported the use of birth control pills (by themselves or their partners) prior to the last sexual intercourse. Furthermore, approximately one fourth (25.6%; female students, 20.7%; male students, 30.9%) had used alcohol or drugs at the time of their last sexual intercourse. Overall, the majority of students (86%; 84% of female students, 89% of male students) reported engaging in responsible sexual behavior, defined as never having sexual intercourse, not engaging in sexual intercourse during the last three months, or using a condom when engaging in sex.

Statistics on adolescent sexual activity (e.g., CDC, 2002b), coupled with prevalence figures for pregnancy and STDs, are cause for concern among researchers and interventionists. For example, the NASP (1997) estimated that almost 1,000 adolescents become pregnant, and 600 contract a venereal disease every day. According to the CDC (2002b), approximately 5% of high school students reported having been pregnant (5.4%) or getting someone pregnant (4%). Concerns over sexual behavior and consequent sexual risks among adolescents have resulted in the development of school-based sexual risk prevention programs focused on pregnancy, HIV/AIDS, and other STDs. The widespread availability of educational programs is illustrated by data from the 2001 YRBSS survey (CDC, 2002b). The vast majority (89%) of high school students nationwide indicated they had received HIV/AIDS education in school.

Rates of pregnancy, birth, and abortion among U.S. adolescents are considered to be among the highest for industrialized nations (Sells & Blum, 1996). In 1999, the birth rate among young women ages 15 to 17 was 29 per 1,000 (a record low for the United States); 88% of these births were to unmarried mothers (compared with 62% in 1980; Federal Interagency Forum on Child and Family Statistics, 2001). The birth rate among adolescents is of particular concern because of short- and long-term difficulties, such as low birth weight, high infant mortality, interruption of the mother's education, and consequences attributable to socioeconomic factors (e.g., poverty, education level, employment status; Federal Interagency Forum on Child and Family Statistics, 2001).

According to the CDC (2001b), adolescents and young adults (ages 10–24) are at higher risk for acquiring STDs, such as chlamydial infection and gonorrhea, than older adults. In 2000, for example, adolescent women and men (ages 15–19) had the highest and third highest rates of gonorrhea in the United States, respectively. The higher prevalence of STDs among adolescents and young adults, compared with older adults, has been attributed to a number of factors, including barriers to health care and prevention services, greater likelihood of engaging in unprotected sexual intercourse, having multiple partners, or selecting high-risk partners (CDC, 2001b). In addition, adolescent women may be more susceptible physiologically to chlamydial infection (CDC, 2001b).

Of particular concern among STDs are HIV (human immunodeficiency virus) infection and AIDS (acquired immunodeficiency syndrome). AIDS has been identified as the sixth leading cause of death among youths (ages 15–24) in the United States, with 20% of all AIDS cases occurring among young adults (ages 20–29) and most acquiring the disease during adolescence (Sells & Blum, 1996). In 1993, the largest annual increase (214%) occurred for adolescents ages 13 to 19 (CDC, 1994).

The CDC has conducted surveillance of HIV/AIDS since the first known cases were reported in the United States in 1981 (CDC, 2000a). The majority of AIDS cases reported to the CDC, both cumulatively from 1981 to December 2000 (99% of 4,467) and for the year 2000 (99.5% of 42,156), were adolescents or adults (i.e., over the age of 13). Of the total cumulative AIDS cases reported to CDC through 2000, 58% are known to have died.

Because of the 10-year latency period from onset of HIV infection to the development of symptomatic AIDS, epidemiological data on AIDS may underestimate the number of adolescents infected with HIV (Gayle, Manoff, & Rogers, 1989). HIV prevalence rates are considered to be a good indicator of recent infections among adolescents "because of the limited time since they began the high-risk behaviors that led to infection" (CDC, 2001a, p. 21). Results from five-year (1993–1997) national surveillance of HIV suggest that prevalence among adolescents and young adults (ages 13–24) are low, ranging from 0.011% for female first-time blood donors (0.027% for males) to 0.4% for patients visiting adolescent hospital- or community-based medicine clinics (which provided family planning, prenatal care, counseling, STD treatment, physical examinations, and general medical care).

Surveillance data from 25 states, collected from January 1996 to June 1999, indicate that youths ages 13 to 24 accounted for a greater proportion of HIV than AIDS cases (13% vs. 3%, respectively; CDC, 2002a). Moreover, despite the decline in AIDS incidence (number of newly diagnosed cases), the number of newly diagnosed HIV cases among youths is not declining (CDC, 2002a).

HIV/AIDS transmission has been attributed to a number of factors. On the basis of reports from the U.S. Department of Health and Human Services, Sells and Blum (1996) identified the leading causes of AIDS transmission for adolescents and young adults (ages 13–24) as sexual contact (male-to-male for males, heterosexual for females) and intravenous drug use. Recent reports from the CDC (2000a) indicate that the primary means of HIV exposure is male-to-male sexual contact for male adolescents or adults, heterosexual contact for female adolescents or adults, and perinatal exposure for pediatric AIDS (children below age of 13). Although injection (intravenous) drug use remains among the leading methods of transmission, the number and proportion of AIDS cases attributed to injecting drugs has declined for women (CDC, 2000a). In the early 1990s, infants of HIV-infected women were identified as the fastest growing group testing seropositive for HIV, with pediatric HIV cases accounting for 2% of all known AIDS cases in the United States (CDC, 1994). More current statistics indicate that pediatric AIDS cases account for 0.5% to 1% of AIDS cases in the United States (CDC, 2000a).

Some researchers have suggested that the prevalence of HIV/AIDS in areas that are economically and socially oppressed is a function of the broader social context surrounding the disease. Steiner (1990) described HIV/AIDS as a "synergism of plagues" and suggested that the high risk among the urban poor is linked to intravenous drug use, racial and ethnic prejudice, high crime or prison rate, and sexual activity among adolescents at younger ages. These "plagues" are exacerbated by the AIDS-related deaths of family members, HIV infection of children (through perinatal transmission), and the psychological and affective difficulties co-occurring or resulting from AIDS among children and adults (Steiner, 1990). Further complicating the lives of the school-age population infected with HIV/AIDS is the stigma and social rejection associated with the disease. In one study, only 51% of 9th- to 12th-grade students who were surveyed thought peers with AIDS should be allowed to attend their school and only 56% were willing to be in class with an HIV-infected peer (Kann et al., 1991). Paradoxically, 91%

of the students surveyed believed they could not be infected by being in class with an HIV-infected student.

Poverty

In addition to the association of social maladies with HIV suggested by Steiner (1990), poverty and adverse socioeconomic conditions have been associated with a host of psychological and social problems. For example, poverty is associated with school difficulties (resulting in retention, expulsion, and dropout), teenage pregnancy, low birth weight and infant mortality, lead poisoning, limited educational attainment, poor employment opportunities and unemployment, and limited emotional support and cognitive stimulation (Children's Defense Fund, 2002; Federal Interagency Forum on Child and Family Statistics, 1997, 2001; Garrison et al., 1999).

Poverty rates in 1999 were the lowest in 20 years, with 16% of children living in poverty (i.e., family income below the poverty threshold; Federal Interagency Forum on Child and Family Statistics, 2001). The likelihood of living in poverty is greater for children living in female-headed households (42% vs. 8% for married couples) and for Black and Hispanic children (33% and 30%, respectively, vs. 9% for White non-Hispanic; Federal Interagency Forum on Child and Family Statistics, 2001).

Diet

Social morbidities related to dietary behaviors also have received attention. According to the NIMH (2001b), the majority of individuals with eating disorders are women. The NIMH (2001b) estimated that 0.5% to 3.7% of females experience anorexia nervosa and 1% to 4.2% experience bulimia during their lifetime, and 2% to 5% of females experience binge-eating disorders in a six-month period. Associated with these eating disorders are illnesses such as depression, anxiety disorders, and substance abuse (NIMH, 2001b). Furthermore, in a 2001 nationwide survey (CDC, 2002b), 29% of adolescents in the general population considered themselves overweight (compared with 10.5% who met the body mass index [BMI] criterion, BMI ≥ 95 percentile by age and sex), and 46% indicated they were trying to lose weight during the preceding 30 days.

Females were significantly more likely than males to report concerns about and efforts to lose weight. Approximately one third (34.9%) of females thought they were overweight (6.9% met the BMI criterion), and 62.3% were trying to lose weight during the preceding 30 days. In comparison, approximately one fourth (23.3%) of males considered themselves overweight (14.2% met BMI criterion), and 28.8% were trying to lose weight. Similarly, high school girls were significantly more likely than their male counterparts to use the following weight control strategies (i.e., to lose weight or avoid gaining weight): (a) exercise (preceding 30 days)—female students, 68.4%; male students, 51%; (b) eating less food, fewer calories, or food low in fat—female students, 58.6%; male students, 28.2%; (c) going without eating for at least 24 hours—female students, 19.1%; male students, 7.6%; (d) taking diet pills, powders, or liquids without a doctor's advice—female students, 12.6%; male students, 5.5%; and (e) vomiting or taking laxatives—female students, 7.8%; male students, 2.9% (CDC, 2002b). Nevertheless, such attitudes and behaviors in both male and female students warrant attention.

Throughout this chapter, discussions of mental health concerns—psychiatric disorders and social morbidities—have focused on the general school-age population. Although prevalence rates often reflect variations by racial, ethnic, and cultural factors, it is beyond the scope of this report to adequately address these variations. The reader is referred to the numerous epidemiological data sources referenced herein for such specificity.[1] The focus on the general population is not meant to minimize the needs of any particular group within the school-age population. Certainly, mental health problems and illness affect all sectors of the United States and global community, although the manifestations may vary with race, ethnicity, gender, age, and culture (USDHHS, 2001a).

The U.S. Surgeon General's report (USDHHS, 2001a) addressed specifically the importance of ethnicity, race, and culture in the promotion of mental health and diagnosis, treatment, and prevention of mental illness within the United States. The Surgeon General's major conclusions deserve the attention of researchers and practitioners devoted to the mental health of children and adolescents. First, culture is a critical variable with regard to the individual's manifestation of symptoms, coping styles, social supports, and use of professional services and the providers' delivery of services. Second, mental disorders are prevalent across all racial and ethnic groups, and prevalence rates among ethnic and racial minority groups are generally similar to those for Whites. The exceptions are (a) vulnerable, high-need groups (e.g., homeless, institutionalized, or incarcerated) who have high prevalence rates and are underrepresented in community surveys, and (b) smaller racial or ethnic minority groups (American Indians, Alaskan Natives, Asian Americans, and Pacific Islanders) who are insufficiently studied. Third, although mental illness is not inherently more serious or more widespread

---

[1]Readers may find reports from the following agencies particularly helpful and can access many of the reports on the respective Web sites: Centers for Disease Control and Prevention (www.cdc.gov); U.S. Department of Health and Human Services, (www.hhs.gov); National Institute of Mental Health (www.nimh.gov); Substance Abuse and Mental Health Services Administration (www.samhsa.gov); Federal Interagency Forum on Child and Family Statistics (www.childstats.gov); and Children's Defense Fund (www.childrensdefense.org).

among minority groups, the burden associated with mental illness is greater because of a number of disparities related to access and availability of high-quality mental health care. Fourth, members of minority groups experience social and economic inequalities (poverty, violence, racism, and discrimination) that influence mental health, the most important of which is poverty. Racism and discrimination represent stressors that can negatively impact mental health. Fifth, specific cultural factors influence the extent to which minorities seek mental health care. These include stigma associated with mental illness, mistrust of providers, and misunderstandings or miscommunications because of cultural differences between patients and providers. The Surgeon General's concerns about access to quality mental health care are shared by others. For example, the NASP (1997) reported that 20% (13.5 million) of children in the United States are living in poverty, and almost 12 million have no health insurance.

In conclusion, the USDHHS (1999) estimated that in a given year, approximately 10% of children and adults receive mental health services in the health sector. Another 5% of adults and 20% of children receive services from other health or mental health care providers in schools, social service agencies, or religious agencies. Although the urgent need for mental health services for children and adolescents in the United States is well documented, factors such as poverty, lack of health insurance, stigma associated with mental illness, and lack of adequate culturally appropriate services are likely to preclude access and use of mental health services for many individuals. With increasing frequency, schools are being called on to resolve problems related to availability of quality mental health care for children and adolescents (Adelman & Taylor, 1998; Nastasi, 2000; Nastasi, Varjas, Bernstein, & Pluymert, 1998a, 1998b; USDHHS, 1999). Psychologists working in schools are well positioned to participate in finding solutions. In the final section of this chapter, we discuss the potential role of school psychologists in the delivery of mental health services.

COMPREHENSIVE MENTAL HEALTH SERVICES

In this section, we provide a concise review of current knowledge regarding delivery of comprehensive mental health services for children and adolescents, with particular attention to factors that characterize effective programming and gaps in current research and practice.[2] This review sets

---

[2] A complete review of the literature on school-based mental health services is beyond the scope of this chapter. The literature relevant to comprehensive programming is vast and encompasses research on prevention, intervention, and treatment for the broad array of difficulties and mediating factors related to mental health problems, psychiatric disorders, and social morbidities. Others have conducted thorough reviews and syntheses that can guide the selection of specific intervention

the stage for consideration of PCSIM as a framework for creating acceptable, effective, and sustainable school-based mental health services.

For the purposes of this discussion, we regard comprehensive mental health services as part of comprehensive health care characterized by an extensive array of services for a broad spectrum of health-related problems, including chronic health or health-related conditions, psychiatric disorders, and social morbidities (Nastasi, 2000, 2004). Comprehensive health programming developed out of recognition of the interrelationships among health, mental health, and education; concerns about the needs of youths, particularly those living in urban communities; and concomitant demands for school and educational reform (Dryfoos, 1993, 1994, 1995). Such efforts were described as a reemergence of school-based services, community action, and school-based health care programs dating back to as early as the turn of the 20th century (Dryfoos, 1993, 1995).

Comprehensive care includes a continuum of services ranging from prevention to treatment for identified health problems and related difficulties (e.g., psychological, social, and educational) in individual and family functioning (Nastasi, 2000, 2004). The scope of services necessitates coordination and integration by multiple providers (e.g., psychological, social service, educational, and medical) across multiple facilities (e.g., schools, social service agencies, clinics, and hospitals). In particular, instituting comprehensive service delivery to children, adolescents, and families requires the merging of public education and public health, and the expansion of professional roles (Klein & Cox, 1995). Indeed, the variety of publication outlets for comprehensive health and mental health literature (e.g., in psychology, education, public health, medicine, and social work journals) reflects its interdisciplinary nature.

During the past decade, numerous comprehensive school- and community-based health and mental health programs have been developed and investigated (Adelman & Taylor, 1998; Attkisson, Dresser, & Rosenblatt, 1995; Behar et al., 1996; DiClemente, Ponton, & Hansen, 1996; Dryfoos, 1994; Klein & Cox, 1995; Knoff, 1996; Kolbe et al., 1997; Ring-Kurtz, Sonnichsen, & Hoover-Dempsey, 1995; Roberts & Hinton-Nelson, 1996;

---

strategies. As we describe the application of PCSIM in subsequent chapters, we make reference to relevant literature. We encourage readers to consult extant reviews of mental health research and practice; in particular, we recommend the following: Catalano, Berglund, Ryan, Lonczak, and Hawkins (1998); DuPaul and Eckert (1997); Durlak and Wells (1997); Greenberg, Domitrovich, and Bumbarger (2000); Hoagwood and Erwin (1997); Hoagwood, Jensen, Petti, and Burns (1996); Howard, Flora, and Griffin (1999); Lonigan, Elbert, and Johnson (1998); Mazza, 1997; Nastasi, Varjas, Bernstein, and Pluymert (1998a, 1998b); National Institute of Mental Health (2001a); National Resource Network for Child and Family Mental Health Services at the Washington Business Group on Health (1999); Nitz (1999); Policy Leadership Cadre for Mental Health in Schools (2001); Prout and Prout (1998); Rones and Hoagwood (2000); Wang, Haertel, and Walberg (1998); Weisz, Donenberg, Han, and Kauneckis (1995).

EXHIBIT 1.2
Critical Components of Effective Comprehensive
School-Based Mental Health Programs

1. Involve integration of educational, mental health, and social services through inter-agency and interdisciplinary collaboration.
2. Focus on the full complement of ecological contexts—school, family, peers, community, society—that influence child and adolescent development and functioning.
3. Provide services that address individual, developmental, and social–cultural factors.
4. Include a full continuum of services, including prevention, risk reduction, early intervention, and treatment.
5. Systematically evaluate program process and outcome.
6. Offer services that are based on empirical evidence of the complex array of factors that influence mental health of children and adolescents.

Note. See Appendix 1.1 for a list of references supporting the inclusion of each of these components.

Weissberg & Elias, 1993). Several components have been identified as critical to effective comprehensive programming (see Exhibit 1.2 and Appendix 1.1; see also Nastasi, 2000, 2004). Effective programs (a) are empirically based; (b) provide a continuum of services from prevention to treatment; (c) address individual and social–cultural factors; (d) involve interdisciplinary and interagency collaboration to address the range of educational, mental health, and social service needs; (e) target the range of ecological contexts that influence children and adolescents; and (f) systematically evaluate program process and outcome. These components are consistent with the public health model of mental health advocated by the U.S. Surgeon General and the USDHHS (1999, 2001a, 2001b). Moreover, the PCSIM is intended to facilitate the development of programs with these characteristics.

Evaluation research generally supports the use of comprehensive programming for promoting the well-being of children and adolescents. In particular, researchers have found comprehensive mental health programs to be acceptable to stakeholders (e.g., families, teachers; Behar et al., 1996; M. Caplan et al., 1992; Dryfoos, 1994, 1995; Saxe, Cross, Lovas, & Gardner, 1995; Walter et al., 1995) and accessible and used by intended recipients (Attkisson et al., 1997; Behar et al., 1996; Dryfoos, 1994, 1995; Hannah & Nichol, 1996; Harold & Harold, 1993; Klein & Cox, 1995; Walter et al., 1995). In addition, feasibility (Attkisson et al., 1997; Cross & Saxe, 1997; Dryfoos, 1994, 1995; Holtzman, 1997; Jordan, 1996; Saxe et al., 1995; Walter et al., 1995) and cost-effectiveness of integrated (vs. fragmented) service delivery have been supported (Dryfoos, 1994, 1995; Jordan, 1996), although findings regarding cost-effectiveness are inconclusive (Behar et al., 1996).

In addition to enhancing access and utilization, comprehensive programs are effective for reducing health and mental health risks and improving the overall functioning of children and adolescents. In particular, research supports the use of comprehensive mental health programs to (a) enhance health-promoting behaviors (e.g., social and emotional competencies; M. Caplan et al., 1992; Cowen et al., 1996; Haynes & Comer, 1996); (b) improve academic and school functioning (Dryfoos, 1994, 1995; Haynes & Comer, 1996; Jordan, 1996; Miller, Brehm, & Whitehouse, 1998); (c) reduce risky behaviors, morbidity, and mortality (M. Caplan et al., 1992; Dryfoos, 1994, 1995; Hannah & Nichol, 1996; Jordan, 1996; Klein & Cox, 1995; Miller et al., 1998; Schoenwald, Henggeler, Pickrel, & Cunningham, 1996); (d) facilitate early identification of high-risk students (Dryfoos, 1994, 1995); and (e) decrease the necessity of restrictive placements (Jordan, 1996).

Although generally supportive of comprehensive school-based services for enhancing individual well-being and reducing risk, research results are not unequivocal (Behar et al., 1996; Kirby et al., 1993; Nastasi & DeZolt, 1994; Nastasi, Varjas, Bernstein, & Pluymert, 1998b; Weissberg, Caplan, & Harwood, 1991). One issue that warrants attention is the extent to which programs can be implemented in a consistent manner by different individuals or in different settings. Within multisite projects, for example, program implementation and evaluation may vary across sites (Attkisson et al., 1997; Cross & Saxe, 1997; Saxe et al., 1995); likewise, perceptions of successful implementation may vary across stakeholders (Attkisson et al., 1997). Such inconsistency in implementation in multisite or replication studies challenges the feasibility of standardizing empirically based programs, as the following comments by Cross and Saxe (1997) suggested:

> That no "right" way exists to develop systems of care, even though the systems share common elements, is not surprising given how dramatically communities differed. . . . The findings from MHSPY [Mental Health Services Program for Youth; 9 sites nationwide] suggest that efforts to develop generic models of systems of care may be misguided and should be viewed skeptically. (p. 67)

Research on organizational change and social program innovations supports such conclusions. McLaughlin (1976, 1990), on the basis of findings from a four-year study of 293 local school-based educational change projects, stated that, "successful implementation [of educational interventions or change projects] is characterized by a process of mutual adaptation" (1976, p. 340). The continual monitoring and modification that characterizes mutual adaptation involve changes in participants (e.g., through staff development) and context (e.g., in classroom structure or practices). Such changes are consistent with the use of context- and culture-specific modifications during implementation in real-life settings (Nastasi, Varjas, Schensul, et al., 2000), a process that is fundamental to program implementation in PCSIM.

EXHIBIT 1.3
Gaps in Comprehensive Mental Health Services

1. Identification of active ingredients, or essential elements, of effective programs
2. Knowledge base to facilitate replication or transfer (i.e., adaptability) of effective programs to other settings and populations
3. Evaluation of unintended outcomes and long-term impact
4. Identification of variables that facilitate or inhibit program implementation
5. Suitability and effectiveness of program for subgroups within the population (i.e., based on gender, ethnicity, race, etc.)
6. Availability of culture-specific evaluation measures
7. Examination of variations or modifications in program implementation, the relationship between modifications and outcomes, and implications for standardization of programs

In addition to issues regarding program adaptations, researchers have identified a number of other gaps in current knowledge about comprehensive programming (see Exhibit 1.3). In particular, further research is needed to address the following issues: (a) adaptation of programs to meet cultural variations within a population (Botvin, Schinke & Orlandi, 1995; Lonigan, Elbert, & Johnson, 1998; Noell, Ary, & Duncan, 1997); (b) development of culture-specific (i.e., appropriate to the values, norms, and language of a specific cultural group) evaluation measures (Nabors, Weist, Holden, & Tashman, 1999); (c) generalization or deployment of evidence-based interventions (studied under highly controlled conditions) to real-life contexts (Evans, 1999; Lonigan et al., 1998; NIMH, 2001a); (d) evaluation of unintended (Wang, Haertel, & Walberg, 1998) and long-term program impact (Arnold, Smith, Harrison, & Springer, 1999); (e) documentation of the active program ingredients (i.e., that account for outcomes), particularly in multicomponent interventions (Knoff & Batsche, 1995; Wang et al., 1998); (f) examination of factors that facilitate or interfere with effective program implementation (Wang et al., 1998); and (g) study of the relationship between variations in implementation (e.g., across service providers) and program outcomes (Eggert, Thompson, Herting, & Nicholas, 1995; Farrell & Meyer, 1997; Wang et al., 1998). Integral to PCSIM are procedures for addressing these gaps.

In conclusion, comprehensive programs are generally acceptable and effective, although critical questions remain regarding active ingredients of multifaceted programs and the deployment of evidence-based interventions. In particular, the individual, contextual, and cultural variations in real-life settings necessitate reconsidering traditional concepts of standardization and experimental control as we attempt to provide effective services in schools and communities. We return to these issues as we describe and illustrate the application of the PCSIM in subsequent chapters.

THE ROLE OF SCHOOL PSYCHOLOGISTS IN
SCHOOL-BASED MENTAL HEALTH SERVICES

The demand for increased participation of schools in meeting the health and mental health needs of students has stemmed from several concerns (Adelman & Taylor, 1998; Nastasi, 2000; Nastasi, Varjas, Bernstein, & Pluymert, 1998b; USDHHS, 1999). First, there is a clear gap between mental health needs and the availability or use of services, especially for poor and minority segments of the population. Second, the link between health or mental health and school performance is well documented. Third, schools have established mechanisms for addressing the needs of special education students, many of whom have unique health or mental health needs. Fourth, the need for comprehensive and coordinated health or mental health services through school- or community-based efforts has been acknowledged. In particular is recognition of the fragmentation and poor coordination of services for children, adolescents, and their families that often lead to ineffective or inadequate prevention, intervention, and treatment efforts. Moreover, schools provide an optimal context for addressing the needs of all students and for the development of school–community–family partnerships.

Psychologists working in schools have traditionally assumed limited roles, primarily focused on conducting diagnostic assessment to determine student eligibility for special education. For several decades school psychologists have been urged to extend those traditional roles to include activities that encompass a broad range of mental health services (Nastasi, 2000; Nastasi, Varjas, Bernstein, & Pluymert, 1998b). Specifically, school psychologists have been encouraged to assume responsibilities as direct service providers for students with mental disorders or at risk for such disorders (Stark, Brookman, & Frazier, 1990) as well as indirect service providers for their families (Christenson, 1995; Garrison et al., 1999); prevention specialists who develop, implement, and evaluate programs to foster mental health promotion or prevention of social morbidities (Elias & Branden, 1988; Nastasi, 2000; Sandoval & Brock, 1996; Talley & Short, 1996); consultants to teachers and administrators regarding classroom-based or building-level mental health services (Curtis & Stollar, 1996; Landau, Pryor, & Haefli, 1995; Paavola et al., 1996); child advocates for school-based services (Doll, 1996; Power, DuPaul, Shapiro, & Parrish, 1995); assessment specialists responsible for developing screening and identification procedures for students at risk for mental health problems (Kolbe et al., 1997; Mazza & Overstreet, 2000); staff developers for school personnel in topics related to mental health promotion and mental health problems or disorders (DeJong, 2000; Landau et al., 1995); and coordinators of systemwide or interagency efforts (Paavola et al., 1996; Pitcher & Poland, 1992; Power, 2000). Coupled with expertise in mental health, school psychologists also have "unique expertise regarding issues of learning in schools" (Sheridan & Gutkin, 2000, p. 488). Thus, they are in a unique position to understand the educational implications of mental health problems and disorders.

Although school psychologists are uniquely qualified as school-based mental health specialists, most of them still spend the majority of their time (reports ranging from over 50% to over 70% of the time) engaged in psychoeducational assessment for the purpose of determining eligibility for special education (Curtis, Hunley, Walker, & Baker, 1999; Reschly, 2000; Reschly & Wilson, 1995). Considerably less time is spent in problem-solving consultation (16%), direct intervention (20%), and organizational consultation or research and evaluation (5% or less; Reschly & Wilson, 1995). Nevertheless, school psychologists have made progress in extending their roles. In one national survey (Curtis et al., 1999), members of the NASP indicated that they engaged in a range of activities. In addition to conducting psychoeducational assessment (reported by 97% of respondents), NASP members engaged in consultation (97%), individual counseling (86%), group counseling (54%), and educational programs for parents, teachers, and others (78%). Similarly, a survey of school psychologists who were members of the American Psychological Association (Short & Rosenthal, 1995) revealed a range of services, including assessment (63% of respondents), consultation (59%), and counseling (64%). Furthermore, respondents to one survey (Reschly & Wilson, 1995) indicated an interest in reallocating time to decrease the amount spent in assessment and increase the amount devoted to other activities such as direct intervention, problem solving and organizational consultation, and research and evaluation.

Studies of school psychologists engaged in delivery of mental health services provided evidence for the realization of an expanded role (Nastasi, Pluymert, Varjas, & Moore, 2002; Nastasi, Varjas, Bernstein, & Pluymert, 1998a). The psychologists who were actively engaged in mental health service provision devoted almost half (48% in 1998; 40% in 2002) of their total work time to development, implementation, and evaluation of a specific mental health program. Most of that time (61% in 1998; 64% in 2002) was spent in program implementation, with the remainder of the time devoted equally to program development and evaluation. In contrast to other surveys, these school psychologists spent less than 30% (21% in 1998; 28% in 2002) of their time in assessment, with the remainder devoted to counseling (20% in 1998; 19% in 2002), consultation (27% in 1998; 24% in 2002), prevention (16% in 1998; 14% in 2002), research (6% in 1998; 5% in 2002), and other activities (9% in 1998 and 2002). In the initial study (Nastasi, Varjas, Bernstein, & Pluymert, 1998a), school psychologists reported using a number of strategies to achieve time reallocation, including modifying assessment and referral practices (e.g., increased use of prereferral teams), delegating responsibilities to other staff, renegotiating roles with administrators, and presenting proposals for mental health programs to administrators. Whereas some psychologists were hired (e.g., through grant money) to work on a specific program, others devoted their own personal time to get a program started. Time allocation and personal initiative proved beneficial for these psychologists. Nevertheless, most school psychologists are still restricted by traditional assessment roles.

Despite the current reality of school psychology practice, what is the potential for involvement in school-based mental health services? Psychologists are being challenged to participate in comprehensive health and mental health care of children and adolescents (Adelman & Taylor, 1998; DeJong, 2000; Kolbe et al., 1997; Kubiszyn, 1999; Nastasi, 2000; Power et al., 1995; Talley & Short, 1996). In addition, psychologists are being urged to expand their practice in ways that have implications for how service provision is conceptualized (Nastasi, 2000). Psychologists are being called on to participate in interdisciplinary health promotion (Leviton, 1996; Stokols, 1992); to provide the full range of services, from prevention to treatment (Nastasi, 1998, 2000); to address the needs of a diverse global and domestic society (Hermans & Kempen, 1998; Nastasi, Varjas, Bernstein, & Jayasena, 2000; Segall, Lonner, & Berry, 1998); to better integrate research and practice (Hoshmand & Polkinghorne, 1992; Nastasi, 1998; Stoner & Green, 1992); and to engage stakeholders as participants in change efforts (Nastasi, Varjas, Bernstein, & Jayasena, 2000; J. J. Schensul, 1998). Together, these demands require a school psychologist with expertise in comprehensive health and mental health care, culturally relevant (or culture-specific) practice, interdisciplinary collaboration, participatory approaches to service provision, and action research methods. This definition is consistent with recently proposed models of psychological practice (DeJong, 2000; Kubiszyn, 1999; Mazza & Overstreet, 2000; Nastasi, 2000; Paavola et al., 1996; Power, 2000; Power et al., 1995; Roberts et al., 1998; Sandoval & Brock, 1996; Sheridan & Gutkin, 2000; Talley & Short, 1996).

Exhibit 1.4 summarizes the key features of the conceptual framework and professional identity of school psychologists serving as health care providers (Nastasi, 2000). These features characterize school-based psychological practice that is consistent with the model of mental health promotion articulated and illustrated in this book. Indeed, the PCSIM is intended to assist school psychologists and other mental health professionals in assuming the role of mental health care provider as outlined in Exhibit 1.4. In chapter 6, we return to the considerations of PCSIM for the practice of psychology in the schools.

EXHIBIT 1.4
School Psychologist as Mental Health Care Provider

Conceptual Framework

View of Person and Environment

- Person and environment are inextricably linked.
- Development is a synergistic process involving continual integration of the individual with context and culture.
- Environment is viewed as ecology, that is, the integration of myriad social–cultural contexts and influences, and the individual's unique interpretation of social–cultural context.
- The focus is the person's overall psychological well-being or mental health.
- The goal is to promote the person's successful life functioning in multiple contexts.

View of Diversity

- Services should be based on in-depth understanding of the individual's culture.
- There are myriad possibilities for healthy functioning.
- Cultural competence implies knowledge about the interaction of cultures of the client, stakeholders, and psychologist.

Professional Identity

School Psychologist as Scientist

- Collaborative and interdisciplinary, integrating psychology, education, medicine, anthropology, sociology, and public health.
- Producer of science.
- Practicing scientist.
- Uses inductive and deductive methods.
- Action researcher.

School Psychologist as Practitioner

- Proactive in social and educational reform.
- Applies interdisciplinary perspective to life functioning in multiple contexts.
- Expert on mental health.
- Integrated roles, encompassing change agent, mental health specialist, systems specialist, advocate, program developer and evaluator, and partner.

Note. From "School Psychologists as Health-Care Providers in the 21st Century: Conceptual Framework, Professional Identity, and Professional Practice," by B. K. Nastasi, 2000, *School Psychology Review, 29,* p. 551. Copyright 2000 by the National Association of School Psychologists. Adapted with permission.

SUMMARY AND CONCLUSIONS

This chapter addressed several key questions: Why are school-based mental health services necessary? What constitutes comprehensive mental health services in schools? How can psychologists contribute to school-based mental health promotion and intervention efforts? The answers to these questions can inform our efforts to develop and enhance school-based mental health services. First, the mental health needs of children and adolescents in the United States have been well documented. Second, the complex interaction of biological, psychological, social, and cultural factors related to mental health requires broad-based interdisciplinary approaches to prevention and treatment. Third, existing evidence supports the effectiveness of comprehensive mental health service delivery systems characterized by a continuum of services, interdisciplinary and interagency collaboration, and the use of ecological and participatory models for program development, implementation, and evaluation. Despite the availability of evidenced-based interventions, questions regarding translation of science to practice prevent effective use of these interventions. In particular, guidelines for adapting interventions across diverse groups and contexts and addressing factors that facilitate or inhibit effective implementation are needed. Finally, the delivery of comprehensive services requires the expertise of mental health professionals working in schools. Psychologists can play a critical role in helping to meet the mental health needs of America's children and adolescents. The presence of school psychologists in districts across the country has not guaranteed their involvement in comprehensive mental health service delivery. Addressing barriers to psychologists' involvement in school-based mental health is critical to the development of effective service delivery.

The remaining chapters are devoted to describing and illustrating a participatory model for creating comprehensive school-based mental health services. In chapter 2, we present the interdisciplinary foundations for the PCSIM. In chapter 3, we introduce and illustrate the components of the model. Chapters 4 and 5 are devoted to in-depth description of the procedures for implementing the PCSIM, with examples from our work and that of others. Chapter 6 concludes the book with discussions of issues related to the use of the PCSIM and future directions for research, training, and practice in school psychology.

APPENDIX 1.1

Critical Components of Comprehensive Mental Health Programs: Supportive Literature

Listed below are the references supporting the inclusion of respective components as fundamental to comprehensive school-based mental health programs (listed in Exhibit 1.2). Readers are encouraged to consult these sources for further information.

1. Integration of educational, mental health, and social services through interagency and interdisciplinary collaboration, for example, through school-based health clinics or school–community systems of care (Adelman & Taylor, 1998; Armbruster & Litchman, 1999; Bickman, 1996; Bickman & Rog, 1995; Borders & Drury, 1992; Flaherty & Weist, 1999; Jennings, Pearson, & Harris, 2000; Klein & Cox, 1995; Nabors et al., 1999; Roberts, 1996; C. A. Smith, 1997; Walter et al., 1995; Wang et al., 1998).

2. Focus on the ecological contexts (i.e., school, family, peers, community, and society) that influence child and adolescent development and functioning:
   - Use a participatory approach to involve stakeholders (e.g., parents, peers, professionals, and teachers) in program decisions to increase acceptability, ownership, social validity, and program integrity (Arnold et al., 1999; Bickman & Rog, 1995; Borders & Drury, 1992; Braswell et al., 1997; Catalano et al., 1998; Cheney, 1998; Cheney & Osher, 1997; Cowen et al., 1996; DiClemente, Ponton, & Hansen, 1996; Flaherty & Weist, 1999; Gottfredson, Fink, Skroban, & Gottfredson, 1997; Kamps & Tankersley, 1996; Kay & Fitzgerald, 1997; Knoff & Batcshe, 1995; Kotkin, 1998; McConaughy, Kay, & Fitzgerald, 1999; McDonald & Sayger, 1998; Moore, Sugland, Blumenthal, Glei, & Snyder, 1995; Nabors, Reynolds, & Weist, 2000; Nelson, Dykman, Powell, & Petty, 1996; Osher & Hanley, 1996; Perry & Kelder, 1992; Ring-Kurtz et al., 1995; Rones & Hoagwood, 2000; S. Smith & Coutinho, 1997; Taylor & Adelman, 2000; Wang et al., 1998).
   - Specifically address ecological or contextual factors (Anglin, Naylor, & Kaplan, 1996; Botvin, Schinke, & Orlandi, 1995; Catalano et al., 1998; Center for Mental Health in Schools, 1997, 1998; deGaston, Jensen, & Weed, 1995; DiClemente,

Ponton, & Hansen, 1996; Dodge, 1993; Dryfoos, 1998; Durlak & Wells, 1997; Farrell & Meyer, 1997; Gresham, 1998; Hoagwood et al., 1996; Roberts, 1996; Rones & Hoagwood, 2000; Schorr, 1997; C. A. Smith, 1997; M. U. Smith & DiClemente, 2000).

3. Provide services that address or adapt to individual, developmental, and social–cultural variations within the target or recipient population (Bickman & Rog, 1995; Botvin, Schinke, & Orlandi, 1995; Clarke et al., 1995; DiClemente, Ponton, & Hansen, 1996; Farrell & Meyer, 1997; Jennings et al., 2000; Kotkin, 1998; National Institute of Mental Health, 2001a; Nitz, 1999; Noell et al., 1997; O'Dea & Abraham, 2000; Perry & Kelder, 1992; Roberts, 1996; Rones & Hoagwood, 2000; M. U. Smith & DiClemente, 2000; Taylor & Adelman, 2000).

4. Provide a broad-based or schoolwide continuum of services, for example, prevention, risk reduction, early intervention, and treatment (Bickman & Rog, 1995; Dadds et al., 1999; DiClemente, Ponton, & Hansen, 1996; Dryfoos, 1995; Eggert et al., 1995; Flaherty & Weist, 1999; Jennings et al., 2000; Knoff & Batsche, 1995; Nabors et al., 1999; Ring-Kurtz et al., 1995; Weist, Myers, Hastings, Ghuman, & Han, 1999).

5. Thorough and systematic program evaluation with the following characteristics: (a) utilizes a multidimensional, multimethod, and multisource approach; (b) assesses process and outcome; (c) integrates intervention and evaluation, for example, by using ongoing assessment to inform adaptations; and (d) considers not only immediate impact but also long-term outcomes and transfer to other settings (Arnold et al., 1999; DiClemente, Ponton, & Hansen, 1996; Eggert et al., 1995; Elias, 1997; Farrell & Meyer, 1997; Gutkin & Curtis, 1999; Hoagwood & Erwin, 1997; Knoff & Batsche, 1995; Kotkin, 1998; McCord, Klein, Foy, & Fothergill, 1993; McDonald & Sayger, 1998; Mortenson & Witt, 1998; Nabors, Reynolds, & Weist, 2000; Nabors, Weist, & Reynolds, 2000; O'Dea & Abraham, 2000; Ring-Kurtz et al., 1995; Roberts, 1996; Wang et al., 1998).

6. Program developed on the basis of theory and empirical evidence regarding the complex array of factors that influence (or mediate) mental health of children and adolescents (Arnold et al., 1999; Bickman & Rog, 1995; Botvin, Schinke, & Orlandi, 1995; Catalano et al., 1998; de Gaston et al., 1995;

DiClemente, Ponton, & Hansen, 1996; Kazdin, Bass, Ayers, & Rodgers, 1990; Lonigan et al., 1998; McDonald & Sayger, 1998; Moore et al., 1995; Nelson et al., 1996; Nitz, 1999; O'Dea & Abraham, 2000; Roberts, 1996; Rones & Hoagwood, 2000; Schinke, 1998; M. U. Smith & DiClemente, 2000).

2

FOUNDATIONS OF THE PARTICIPATORY CULTURE-SPECIFIC INTERVENTION MODEL

In this chapter, we provide an overview of the foundations of the participatory culture-specific intervention model (PCSIM). The PCSIM is an interdisciplinary model grounded in concepts, methods, and procedures from the fields of applied anthropology and school psychology. Contributions from these two fields help to extend traditional models of program development. The seeming simplicity of the traditional model, depicted in Figure 2.1, is deceiving given the complexity and dynamic nature of school-based intervention. We propose that the participatory intervention model, depicted in Figure 2.2, more clearly reflects the reality of program development.

Participatory and traditional program development models differ in four important ways. First, traditional models are typically depicted as a linear progression from program design to implementation to evaluation (see Figure 2.1), whereas participatory models reflect a more fluid and recursive process in which program developers are continuously engaged in decision making about and reconsideration of design, implementation, and evaluation activities (see Figure 2.2). This recursive process more accurately depicts the reality of conducting interventions in real-life settings, in which conditions and players are dynamic, thus necessitating monitoring (evaluation) of and adaptations to (redesign of) the intervention. Second,

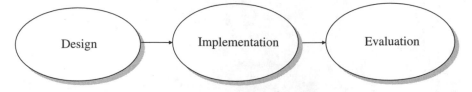

Figure 2.1. Traditional intervention model: The three phases—design, implementation, and evaluation—are traditionally viewed as steps of a linear process carried out by intervention experts. The simplicity of the design masks the underlying complexity.

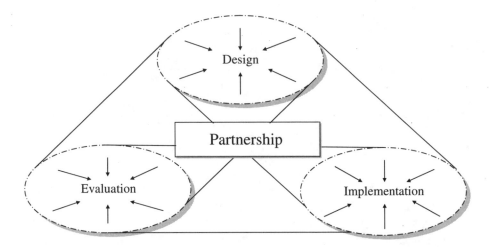

Figure 2.2. Participatory intervention model: In contrast to the linear nature of the traditional intervention model depicted in Figure 2.1, the participatory model involves a recursive process of program design, implementation, and evaluation. In addition, partnership among program planners, interventionists, evaluators, and other stakeholders is central to the intervention process. From "Participatory Model of Mental Health Programming: Lessons Learned From Work in a Developing Country," by B. K. Nastasi, K. Varjas, S. Sarkar, and A. Jayasena, 1998, *School Psychology Review, 27,* p. 261. Copyright 1998 by the National Association of School Psychologists. Adapted with permission. (See also Nastasi, Varjas, Schensul, et al., 2000.)

traditional models are typically expert-oriented, with the program developer guiding the process and stakeholders viewed as recipients of the program. In contrast, stakeholders in participatory models are viewed as partners throughout program development, and partnership is viewed as central to the participatory intervention process (see Figure 2.2). Third, traditional approaches to program development do not necessarily attend to culture-specific aspects, a critical element in participatory models such as PCSIM. Fourth, traditional models are not inherently interdisciplinary, in contrast to the necessary interdisciplinary focus of participatory models such as PCSIM. Indeed, the transition in our own work from traditional intervention approaches to a participatory culture-specific approach was facilitated by interdisciplinary collaboration and integration of research and practice methods from psychology and anthropology.

The four foundational components of PCSIM—*participatory action research, participatory culture-specific consultation, ecological perspective*, and *ethnography*—provide the conceptual, methodological, and procedural bases for development, implementation, and evaluation of interventions, specifically school-based mental health programs. The PCSIM is grounded conceptually in ecological–developmental theory (Bronfenbrenner, 1989), methodologically in action research and ethnography, and procedurally in participatory culture-specific consultation. We describe each foundational component, its link to the practice of psychology in schools, and its contribution to PCSIM. Much has been written about each of these components. We provide here an overview and suggest that readers consult the respective referenced sources for more comprehensive treatment of these topics.

PARTICIPATORY ACTION RESEARCH

Action research corresponds to the data-based problem-solving approach of school psychology, in which a research (data gathering and interpreting) process guides decisions about intervention or practice (Nastasi, 1998). Participatory action research (PAR) corresponds to the collaborative data-based problem-solving approach in which psychologists work with other school personnel (e.g., teachers, administrators) and parents to make decisions about interventions for specific students.

Action research and PAR have roots in applied anthropology (Greenwood, Whyte, & Harkavy, 1993; Nastasi, 1998; J. J. Schensul, 1998; J. J. Schensul & Schensul, 1992) and involve a recursive process linking theory, research, and practice to foster social and cultural change. The process of action research (Figure 2.3) is initiated with formative research, driven by the research question, and informed by existing research and theory. Formative research findings provide the generative basis for designing culture- or context-specific (local) theory (i.e., theory that accounts for natural phenomena in the target context and population). This local theory then provides the basis for design of the culture or context-specific (local) intervention or action. Evaluation of the intervention, through research, informs not only adaptations of the intervention but also development of general and culture-specific theory, thus adding to the existing personal knowledge

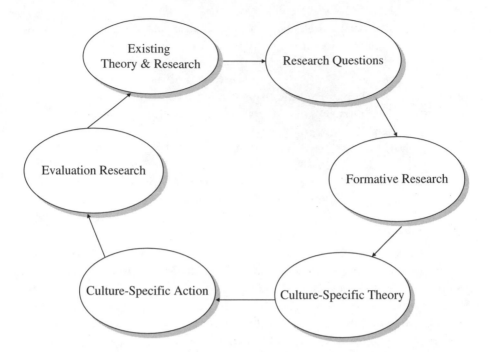

Figure 2.3. Action research process: Action research is characterized by a recursive process that involves (a) the use of existing theory and research, (b) generation of research questions, (c) conducting formative research to (d) develop culture-specific (local) theory and (e) action, and (f) evaluation that subsequently influences extant theory and research knowledge. From "A Model for Mental Health Programming in Schools and Communities," by B. K. Nastasi, 1998, *School Psychology Review, 27,* p. 170. Copyright 1998 by the National Association of School Psychologists. Adapted with permission.

of the practitioner and potentially to scientific knowledge more generally (e.g., through presentations and publications). Participatory Action Research is characterized by the involvement of key stakeholders (i.e., those with relevant interest or resources) as partners in this recursive action research process. Thus, stakeholders participate in decision making and activities of the research-intervention process. The PCSIM is an adaptation of PAR, resulting from the integration of the action research process with the phases of program development. Consistent with its origins in applied anthropology, interventions (e.g., mental health programs) generated using PCSIM are viewed as efforts in social–cultural as well as individual change.

Applied to the development of interventions in schools, action research within PCSIM provides "a systematic way to apply the scientific method to school psychology practice and to make explicit the integration of theory, research, and practice" (Nastasi, 2000, p. 543). Such practice is consistent with the notion of the school psychologist as *reflective practitioner,* who goes beyond the mere application of existing theory and research to active engagement in intervention as a research process (Nastasi, 1998).

PARTICIPATORY CONSULTATION

Participatory consultation refers to a process of consensus building and negotiation of divergent ideas leading to the co-construction of change efforts by researchers–interventionists and stakeholders working in partnership (Nastasi, Varjas, Bernstein, & Jayasena, 2000). The process of engaging stakeholders in program development (i.e., in the application of PAR) is similar to that of collaborative or participatory consultation models for the delivery of school psychological services (Christenson & Conoley, 1992; Nastasi, Varjas, Bernstein, & Jayasena, 2000; Nastasi, Varjas, Schensul, et al., 2000; Rosenfield & Gravois, 1996; Sheridan, Kratochwill, & Bergan, 1996).

In participatory consultation, the interventionists (consultants) engage in a series of formal and informal interactions with key stakeholders (e.g., teachers, parents, administrators) to identify problems and design and evaluate relevant interventions. In practice, consultants working with stakeholders vary along a continuum from expert to equal partner (Nastasi, Varjas, Schensul, et al., 2000). For example, consultants using traditional approaches assume a more expert (prescriptive) role, in which they have authority over decisions about intervention and control the intervention process (Graham, 1998; Wickstrom, Jones, LaFleur, & Witt, 1998). In these instances, consultants attempt to design programs that stakeholders (consumers) will find acceptable, recognizing that interventions that are not acceptable are unlikely to be used or implemented with integrity, and thus unlikely to be effective (Elliott, Witt, & Kratochwill, 1991).

Using a collaborative (or participatory[1]) model, consultants engage stakeholders as full partners in the process of designing, implementing, and evaluating interventions to address identified problems (cf. Graham, 1998; Greenwood et al., 1993; Wickstrom et al., 1998). The level of involvement

---

[1]*Collaboration* and *participation* are often used interchangeably to indicate active involvement of recipients of interventions (in traditional vernacular, "clients") or the researched ("the subjects") in the process of intervention or applied research. Both terms imply horizontal rather than hierarchical (expert) relationships between the interventionists–researchers and the recipients or researched. Serrano-Garcia (1990, p. 174) drew the following distinction with reference to community research: "*Collaboration* . . . denotes engaging the researched in executing the research; whereas *participation* entails their full involvement . . . in planning, decision making, and execution of tasks in the research process." Consistent with this distinction, we prefer the term *participatory* to describe the consultation or intervention process in which recipients or consumers are involved as equal partners with consultants–interventionists throughout the process of design, implementation, and evaluation, with the goal of promoting ownership, sustainability, and institutionalization.

is expected to enhance acceptability and ownership of interventions by stakeholders (Nastasi, Varjas, Schensul, et al., 2000). Although full involvement is the goal of participatory consultation, the actual contribution of stakeholders is likely to vary as a function of contextual factors (e.g., resources, organizational structure) and the motivation and competencies of participants (Greenwood et al., 1993).

Building on contemporary models of scientifically based school psychology (Gutkin & Curtis, 1999; Kratochwill & Stoiber, 2000; Stoiber & Kratochwill, 2000; Stoner & Green, 1992), program evaluation (Fetterman, 1994; Illback, Zins, & Maher, 1999), organizational development (Blakely et al., 1987; McLaughlin, 1976, 1990; Weissberg, 1990), community capacity-building (Eade, 1997), and PAR, we have proposed a participatory culture-specific approach to consultation that parallels the aforementioned participatory intervention model and formed the basis for development of PCSIM. The integration of action research and collaborative consultation results in a recursive series of nine steps depicted in Figure 2.4. In participatory culture-specific consultation (PCSC), stakeholders and consultants work as partners to identify and define problems, collect data, and develop culture-specific explanations of naturally occurring phenomena relevant to the target issue. The culture-specific explanation then guides design of the intervention. The key additions in PCSC to action research (depicted in Figure 2.3) are phases specifically devoted to learning the culture, forming partnerships, and institutionalization of change efforts (shaded areas of Figure 2.4). (For a more in-depth discussion of PCSC, see Nastasi, Varjas, Bernstein, & Jayasena, 2000.) The participatory process inherent in PCSC reflects our approach to inclusion of stakeholders as partners in PCSIM.

ECOLOGICAL PERSPECTIVE

The documented role of family, peer group, school, community, and society in promoting the mental health of children and adolescents (Bickman & Rog, 1995; Hawkins, Catalano, & Miller, 1992; NIMH, 2001a; Roberts, 1996; see chap. 1, this volume) necessitates an ecological perspective (e.g., Bronfenbrenner, 1989). As depicted in Figure 2.5, the ecology of the child or adolescent is complex, involving the interaction of the multiple contexts (ecosystems; e.g., home, school, peer group, community) in which the child or adolescent functions. According to ecological–development theory (Bronfenbrenner, 1989), a person's functioning reflects the ongoing mutual accommodation of the person and the ecology in which he or she lives. The individual (e.g., a student; Figure 2.6) is influenced not only directly by interactions with the immediate context (microsystem; e.g., classroom) but also indirectly by the broader structural context (exosystem; e.g., school)

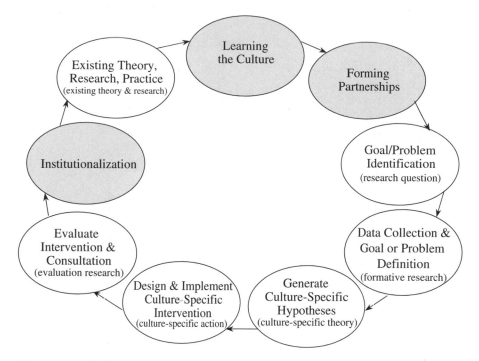

Figure 2.4. Participatory culture-specific consultation: The integration of action research (Figure 2.3) and collaborative consultation results in a recursive series of nine steps depicted here. Note the addition of three (shaded) phases: Learning the Culture, Forming Partnerships, and Institutionalization. From "Conducting Participatory Culture-Specific Consultation: A Global Perspective on Multicultural Consultation," by B. K. Nastasi, K. Varjas, R. Bernstein, and A. Jayasena, 2000, *School Psychology Review, 29,* p. 404. Copyright 2000 by the National Association of School Psychologists. Adapted with permission.

and societal or cultural values, beliefs, and norms or laws that influence the exosystem (macrosystem; e.g., cultural values and norms that influence public education). Moreover, interactions within a given ecosystem are also influenced by interactions between ecosystems (mesosystems; e.g., school–home, family–peer group, or family–school–community). Understanding an individual's mental health status at any given point in time thus requires consideration of current and past interactions within and across the multiple ecosystems. Add to this picture the exponential complexity due to the cultural experiences of other key players (teachers, school administrator, other students, parents, peers, etc.) and the challenge of understanding and influencing the mental health of an individual student becomes evident.

Consideration of the child's or adolescent's ecology has important implications for psychologists working in schools and, more specifically, for the development of school-based mental health programs. Assessment of mental health concerns, for example, requires examining the individual's

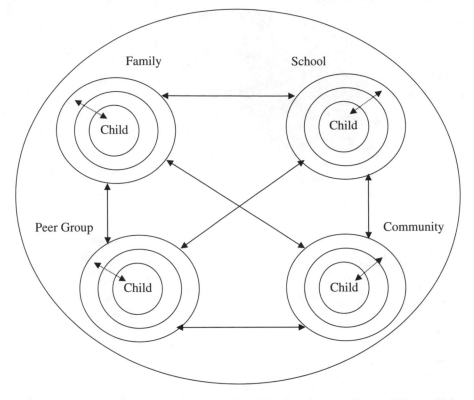

Figure 2.5. The ecology of the child: The child functions or lives within multiple interacting ecosystems of family, school, peer group, and community. Understanding the influences of these multiple systems is critical to mental health assessment and intervention.

functioning within each of the relevant ecosystems (e.g., school, home, community, peer group) and the potential contributions of key socializing agents (e.g., parents, siblings, peers, school personnel). Intervention efforts directed toward the individual child or adolescent are likely to involve one or more of the key players as agents of change. Moreover, changes in the individual's functioning are likely to have an impact on existing ecosystems and socializing agents. Finally, given the essential role of key stakeholders as socializing agents, their involvement in programming is critical to the sustainability and institutionalization of interventions.

The importance of an ecological perspective is well recognized within school psychology, as exemplified in efforts to foster school–family collaboration (Christenson & Buerkle, 1999; Christenson & Conoley, 1992; Sheridan, Kratochwill, & Bergan, 1996); multicultural, ecological, and systemic–organizational approaches to consultation (Borgelt & Conoley, 1999; Curtis

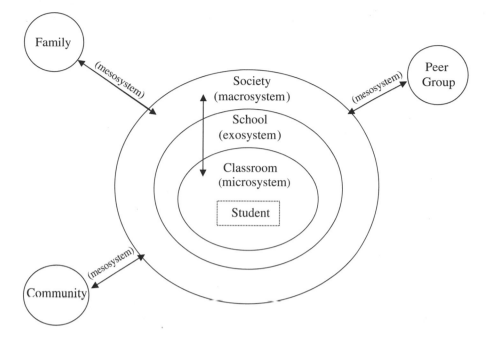

Figure 2.6. Components of the child's ecosystem: The ecological system of the child (student) includes (a) *microsystem* (e.g., classroom), the immediate context; (b) *exosystem* (e.g., school), the broader structural context that encompasses the microsystem; (c) *macrosystem* (e.g., related to public education), the societal or cultural beliefs, values, norms or laws that influence the exosystem; and (d) *mesosystem* (e.g., between school and home), the interaction between ecosystems. This depiction is based on Bronfenbrenner's (1989) ecological–developmental theory.

& Stollar, 1996; Gutkin & Curtis, 1999; Ingraham, 2000); ecologically based intervention approaches (Nastasi & DeZolt, 1994); attention to contextual factors in assessment (Sheridan & Walker, 1999; Ysseldyke & Christenson, 2002; Ysseldyke & Elliott, 1999); and use of an ecological paradigm to conceptualize school psychology practice (Sheridan & Gutkin, 2000). Despite these efforts, researchers, practitioners, the public, and public officials continue to call for greater attention to cultural and ecological factors.

The significance of the ecological perspective is also reflected in the centrality of culture specificity in the PCSIM. Attention to culture specificity is ensured through the participation of stakeholders as ecological informants and change agents, and the use of ethnography for systematic investigation of contextual and cultural factors. In the next section, we discuss ethnography as a methodological foundation of PCSIM and as a mechanism for extending traditional psychological assessment and intervention approaches.

ETHNOGRAPHY

Essential to PCSIM is a process of disciplined inquiry that makes use of qualitative or naturalistic research methods, specifically ethnography, for developing and evaluating interventions (Nastasi & Berg, 1999; Nastasi, Varjas, Schensul, et al., 2000; J. J. Schensul & LeCompte, 1999; Spradley, 1979, 1980).[2] Ethnographic inquiry is conducted in real-life settings and yields in-depth and idiographic representation of phenomena from the perspective of the population the researcher is studying. Such inquiry can assist mental health researchers and interventionists in developing culture- and context-specific programs. The process of ethnographic inquiry is iterative, thus facilitating natural adaptation (modification) of programs to the needs of specific individuals and settings. Because ethnography is devoted to the study of culture, it is particularly well suited for work with multicultural populations in the United States and for extending work to other countries.

Consistent with a recent report by the U.S. Surgeon General (USDHHS, 2001a[3]), we adopt a broad conception of *culture specificity* that extends beyond racial, ethnic, and linguistic specificity:

> Culture specificity implies that critical elements of the intervention (e.g., intervention strategies and targeted competencies) are relevant to the targeted culture, make use of the language of the population, and reflect the values and beliefs of members of the culture. Inherent in this model is the assumption that one cannot separate person from culture and that understanding the culture is essential to understanding the individual. In addition, change efforts cannot be solely person-centered, but must address the role of culture in promoting and sustaining behavior patterns. (Nastasi, 1998, p. 169)

In this conception of culture specificity, we define *culture* as the beliefs, values, language, ideas, and behavioral norms shared by the members of the

---

[2]Other recommended sources on naturalistic–qualitative–ethnographic inquiry include Bernard (1995), Creswell (1997), Denzin and Lincoln (2000), Lincoln and Guba (1985), Miles and Huberman (1994), Ryan and Bernard (2000), Strauss and Corbin (1990), and Wolcott (1994).
[3]The U.S. Surgeon General (USDHHS, 2001a) recommended development of culture-specific approaches to mental health programming that extend beyond development of targeted interventions for specific racial or ethnic groups. His recommendations included consideration of social influences on mental health and mental health care, and, more important, the cultural background of both the client–patient and provider–clinician. In addition, the Surgeon General's call for attention to cultural competence of service providers is consistent with guidelines of the American Psychological Association (1993) for working with culturally, ethnically, and linguistically diverse populations. Responding to the Surgeon General's recommendations requires rethinking our current approaches to mental health services and brings into question the application of standard programs that are designed and marketed for universal use. Moreover, cultural variations may necessitate the development and validation of culture-specific assessment tools for screening, identification, and program evaluation.

culture. Consistent with an ecological view, understanding the culture of the individuals requires consideration of not only their cultural experiences but also their interpretations of those experiences. Appreciating a person's cultural background thus entails awareness of the myriad cultural experiences, interpretations of those experiences, and multiplicity of ecological contexts relevant to that person's life. Furthermore, the cultural diversity within any school or classroom necessitates consideration of both shared and unique cultural experiences of the students, teachers, and other relevant socializing agents.

The characteristics of naturalistic (and ethnographic) inquiry identified by Lincoln and Guba (1985) are relevant to PCSIM foundations and practices, as depicted in Table 2.1. Moreover, the methods of naturalistic inquiry are consistent with those used by school psychologists in practice (e.g., observations, interviews, records review) and thus represent an extension, rather than replacement, of the techniques germane to psychologists working in school settings. By reframing these less formalized components of data collection associated with psychological practice as a formal system of applied ethnographic research, we hope to contribute to narrowing the schism between intervention research and practice (Nastasi, 1998).

In-depth discussion of qualitative inquiry and its methods is beyond the scope of this chapter. We restrict our coverage to an overview of ethnographic methods for data collection, analysis and interpretation, and the criteria and techniques for ensuring trustworthiness (reliability, validity) of findings. Readers are encouraged to consult the aforementioned sources for further information.

Data Collection

Ethnographic data collection techniques include participant observation, key-informant and in-depth interviews, focus groups, collection of artifacts (e.g., permanent products), journals or activity logs, ethnographic surveys, pilesorts, and listing techniques (Table 2.2). These techniques can be used in PCSIM to conduct formative research during program design, to monitor program implementation and guide adaptation, and to evaluate program acceptability, integrity, social validity, outcomes, sustainability, and institutionalization. As we describe the application of PCSIM to developing comprehensive school-based mental health programs in subsequent chapters, we illustrate the use of ethnographic methods in respective phases. These methods are particularly critical during formative research and evaluation phases. (For a more in-depth discussion and illustration of the application of ethnographic methods to program development and evaluation, see Nastasi & Berg, 1999.)

TABLE 2.1
Characteristics of Ethnographic (Naturalistic) Inquiry

Characteristic	Description (Lincoln & Guba, 1985)	Relevance to other PCSIM foundations	Relevance to PCSIM practices
Natural setting	Inquiry is conducted in real-life settings; findings are context- or culture-bound.	Ecological perspective implies attention to real-life culture and context.	Adaptations to culture and context are critical.
Human instrument	Researcher is primary data-collection instrument. Researcher's relationship skills are critical.	Interpersonal relationships and partnerships are critical in PAR and PCSC.	Interpersonal skills are critical to negotiation of partnerships and negotiations of meaning with stakeholders. Program developer is viewed as "human instrument."
Use of tacit knowledge	Influence of researcher's implicit knowledge on research process warrants consideration and documentation.	Use of tacit knowledge is consistent with the reflective nature of scientist–practitioner.	Existing theory, research, and practice influence the researcher's perspective and are reflected in "personal theory" that guides program development.
Qualitative methods	Uses methods that capture natural phenomena and relies primarily on narrative observation and in-depth interviewing. Qualitative methods do not preclude the use of quantitative methods.	Qualitative methods are similar to observation, interviewing, and records review used in professional psychological practice.	Ethnographic methods are used in formative and evaluative research to capture natural phenomena and cultural meaning and to ensure culture specificity.
Purposive sampling	Participant (sample) selection is dependent on research question or focus, to best represent natural phenomena and cultural meaning. Sampling is not necessarily random or focused on normative perspective.	Purposive sampling is consistent with emergent and recursive design of PAR and PCSC, and purposive sampling of psychological practice.	Participant (sample) selection is dependent on focus or purpose of intervention. Sampling strategies vary across PCSIM phases (e.g., formative vs. evaluative).

Inductive data analysis	Meaning is generated from data collected in the natural setting and reflects emic[a] perspective. Hypotheses, themes, and conceptual models emerge from the data.	PCSC involves the negotiation of etic[b] and emic perspectives.	Development of interventions involves integration of emic and etic perspectives. Incorporation of emic view helps to achieve culture specificity.
Grounded theory	Theory emerges empirically from (is grounded in) data, to represent what happens naturally. Research is not driven by a priori theory, and requires clear articulation of researcher's biases.	A primary objective of both PAR and PCSC is to represent emic perspective. In practice, the participatory process is likely to result in the blending of emic and etic perspectives.	Grounded theory is critical to developing culture-specific or local theory and interventions. In practice, culture-specific theory is integration of emic and etic perspectives.
Emergent design	Design emerges from recursive process of data collection, analysis, and interpretation; and requires in-depth documentation of research process.	Emergent process and data-based decision making are inherent in PAR and PCSC.	Development and adaptation of culture- and context-specific interventions reflect emergent design (i.e., research drives intervention decisions).
Negotiated outcomes	Researcher and participants negotiate the meaning or interpretation of data to ensure that findings reflect participant perspective.	Participatory process, inherent in PAR and PCSC, involves negotiation of meaning and joint decision making.	Negotiated meaning is critical to promoting acceptability, ownership, and culture specificity. Participatory process is mechanism for ensuring negotiated meaning.
Case study reporting	In-depth contextualized report, or thick description, reflects idiographic focus and emphasis on contextual specificity and is critical to transferability of findings.	Case study (idiographic vs. nomothetic) is the mode of PAR, PCSC, and psychological, clinical, and school practice.	In-depth documentation and thick description of intervention provides detail for practitioners interested in transferability, thereby helping to bridge research–practice gap.
Idiographic interpretation	Interpretation of findings is restricted to specific sample and setting; reflects particular and contextualized nature of natural phenomena; and facilitates decision making about transferability.	Applied work (practice) in psychology (e.g., PCSC); requires idiographic interpretation. Ecological perspective necessitates recognition of myriad personal and environmental factors related to psychological functioning.	Effective interventions require recognition of complexity of natural phenomena and individual, cultural, and contextual specificity. Adaptation of interventions to individual and contextual variations is crucial.

(continued)

TABLE 2.1 (Continued)

Characteristic	Description (Lincoln & Guba, 1985)	Relevance to other PCSIM foundations	Relevance to PCSIM practices
Tentative application	Conditional nature of findings is recognized, and reader is cautioned about application to other individuals, groups, or settings without further inquiry. Decisions about transferability are considered the responsibility of the consumer.	Data-based problem solving within psychology (e.g., PCSC) requires formulation of interventions based on particulars of the case. The specificity of interventions to individual and context are recognized in both action research and ecological perspective.	Conditional nature of intervention effectiveness (dependent on personal, cultural, and contextual factors) is assumed. PCSIM provides process for transfer of interventions to other individuals, cultures, and contexts.
Focus-determined boundaries	Decisions about parameters of inquiry are based on the purpose, question, or problem being researched. Despite inductive, open-ended nature of inquiry, work is bounded by specific focus. Emergent design requires continual attention to focus.	Parameters of PAR, PCSC, and other psychological practices depend on problem or question being addressed. Parameters change as function of changing focus (e.g., problem definition). Ecological perspective permits consideration of dynamic interaction of individual, cultural, and contextual factors.	Parameters of PCSIM research-intervention process are determined by target problem, needs, and resources of stakeholders. Focus and parameters are continually open to reformulation by partners to meet dynamic individual and contextual factors.
Special criteria for trustworthiness	These criteria for data collection, analysis, and interpretation are intended to ensure reliable and valid findings. Researchers are expected to engage in prolonged and in-depth study; integrate data from multiple methods, sources, and perspectives; confirm the veracity of data and interpretations with stakeholders; and describe procedures in detail.	These criteria are applicable to PAR and PCSC, and consistent with professional conduct of school psychological practice.	Criteria for trustworthiness are inherent in the process and procedures of PCSIM.

Note. See also Lincoln and Guba (1985) for detailed discussion. PCSIM = participatory culture-specific intervention model; PAR = participatory action research; PCSC = participatory culture-specific consultation.
[a]Emic refers to the "insider's" viewpoint, for example, that of the stakeholder, client, consultee. [b]Etic refers to the "outsider's" viewpoint, for example, that of the researcher, interventionist, consultant.

TABLE 2.2
Ethnographic Data Collection Techniques

Technique	Definition	School-based example
Key-informant interview	Informal, unstructured interview or discussion with knowledgeable key stakeholders	Informal discussion with knowledgeable teacher about discipline problems in the school
In-depth interview	Formal, semistructured interview with purposive or random sample of key stakeholders	Interviews with sample of teachers about discipline problems they encounter
Focus group	Formal, semistructured interview with group of key stakeholders, chosen purposefully or randomly	Group interview with six to eight teachers about discipline concerns and strategies
Participant (naturalistic) observation	Narrative (or videotaped) observation in real-life context; level of participation can vary from non- to full participation	In-depth narrative recording of teacher–student interactions in classroom
Ethnographic survey	"Culture-specific" instrument developed based on formative ethnographic data, for purpose of gathering data from larger purposive/random sample	Teacher-report instrument of discipline concerns and techniques, with content derived from in-depth interviews and participant observations
Freelist	Participants asked to list items/examples for a specific domain; the most common items are then used for pilesorting	Teachers are asked to list all the discipline strategies that come to mind
Pilesort	Participants asked to sort cards with/without guidelines for sorting (The purpose of freelist or pilesort techniques is to elicit understanding—definitions of key concepts from the perspective of cultural members.)	Teachers are asked to sort cards reflecting various discipline strategies without guidelines, or relative to severity of discipline problems
Fieldnotes	Narrative record of informal contacts, observations, impressions, and so on	Psychologist's record of all contacts and observations relevant to discipline in the school
Journal/log	Written records of participants; to document activities, reactions, and so on	Teachers asked to record how discipline problems are handled over a one-week period
Artifact	Tangible products	Schoolwide record of suspensions and expulsions
Social network	Spatial–graphic depiction of interpersonal relationships or interactions within specific group or context	Nature and frequency of contacts among service providers; friendship networks within a classroom
Spatial mapping	Spatial–graphic depiction of people, places, objects, or activity within specific geographic context	Spatial organization of the classroom; location of violence incidents within a school building

Data Analysis and Interpretation

The task of organizing, analyzing, and interpreting qualitative data can be overwhelming. The open-ended nature of ethnographic data collection results in vast amounts of raw data, most frequently in the form of notes and text. Yet, the process of transforming data through description, analysis, and interpretation is fundamental to qualitative inquiry (Wolcott, 1994).[4] Making sense of (or transforming) data depends on both the technical and conceptual skills of the researcher. Just as with data collection, the researcher also is the primary instrument for analysis and interpretation. This does not mean that the sense-making process is unsystematic. On the contrary, the generation of trustworthy (i.e., credible, dependable, transferable, and confirmable) findings requires meticulous and methodical management and transformation of the data. Several principles for data transformation and their relevance to PCSIM and to psychological practice in schools are depicted in Table 2.3. (A full treatment of data management, analysis, and interpretation procedures is beyond the scope of this section. Readers are encouraged to consult several excellent sources: LeCompte & Schensul, 1999; Miles & Huberman, 1994; Ryan & Bernard, 2000; Wolcott, 1994.)

Ensuring Trustworthiness

Special criteria and procedures for data collection, analysis, and interpretation proposed by Lincoln and Guba (1985) are essential for establishing the trustworthiness of qualitative findings. These criteria—credibility, transferability, dependability, and confirmability—parallel the requirements of internal validity, external validity, reliability, and objectivity, respectively, in traditional research (Lincoln & Guba, 1985)[5]:

1. *Credibility* refers to the extent to which findings and interpretations are plausible (i.e., acceptable) to the research participants.
2. *Transferability* refers to the applicability of findings to other situations based on comparability with the research context.

---

[4] We adopt Wolcott's (1994) nomenclature for the transformation process—description, analysis, and interpretation:

> *Description* addresses the question, "What is going on here?" Data consist of observations made by the researcher and/or reported to the researcher by others. *Analysis* addresses the identification of essential features and the systematic description of relationships among them—in short, how things work. . . . [When there are stated objectives, for example, in evaluative research] analysis also may be employed evaluatively to address questions of why the system is not working or how it might be made to work "better." *Interpretation* addresses processual questions of meanings and contexts: "[What] does it all mean?" "What is to be made of it all?" (Wolcott, 1994, p. 12)

[5] See also S. L. Schensul, Schensul, and LeCompte (1999) for discussion of reliability and validity issues in ethnographic research.

TABLE 2.3

Principles of Ethnographic Data Transformation: Relevance to Participatory Culture-Specific Intervention Model (PCSIM) and Psychological Practice

Principle	Relevance to PCSIM	Relevance to school psychological practice
1. Data transformation is ongoing and recursive.	Continual research–practice integration	Ongoing nature of data-based decision making
2. Data transformation involves the integration of emic and etic perspectives.	Stakeholders as partners in data analysis and interpretation	Stakeholder involvement in data-based decision making
3. Systematic documentation of procedures is essential.	In-depth documentation of procedures	Record keeping
4. Use both descriptive and inferential language in reports.	Cultural/contextual specificity of findings	Link inferences to descriptive data, to enhance understanding
5. Maximize data triangulation and mixed methodology.	Findings reflect multiple perspectives and multiple sources of data	Multimethod, multisource, multidisciplinary approaches
6. Search for confirming and disconfirming evidence.	Application/adaptation to individual, cultural, and contextual variations is critical	Search for consistencies and discrepancies across contexts, data sources, methods, and so on
7. Make interpretation specific to purpose and audience for dissemination.	Findings presented to varied professional and lay stakeholder groups	Findings presented to different stakeholders (e.g., child, parent, school staff)
8. Data transformation is a participatory process.	Stakeholders as partners throughout the PCSIM process	Participatory approaches to consultation; team process for decision making

3. *Dependability* refers to the extent to which researchers have accounted for factors of instability and change in the natural context.
4. *Confirmability* refers to the capacity to authenticate the internal coherence of data, findings, interpretations, and recommendations.

Researchers and interventionists using PCSIM are expected also to make use of trustworthiness procedures recommended by Lincoln and Guba (1985; defined in Table 2.4). Thus, in designing, implementing, and evaluating an intervention, they are expected to spend a sufficient amount of time in the target setting and with stakeholders to build rapport, correct misinformation, and learn the culture or context (*prolonged engagement*). In addition, an in-depth and clearly focused understanding of the problem and contributing factors requires *persistent observation* in the target context. *Triangulation* of data sources (e.g., stakeholders), methods (observation, interview, self-report, archives), and investigators (e.g., professional staff) is consistent with the multisource, multimethod, and multidisciplinary approach that characterizes both PCSIM and school psychology practice. The interdisciplinary nature of PCSIM provides opportunities for discussing alternative interpretations of data (*peer debriefing*). Continual *member checks* (i.e., verifying data, interpretations, and recommendations with stakeholders) are a necessary part of a participatory approach to intervention programming and are consistent with psychological practice in which clients and significant others are consulted about the veracity of findings. Case study reporting necessitates *thick description* of context. The concept of *audit trail* is consistent with careful record keeping (of raw data, data analysis, and interpretation) that characterizes accountability in PCSIM specifically, and school psychological practice more generally. *Negative case analysis* (consideration of the atypical) is beneficial to a complete understanding of the limits of intervention acceptability, integrity, and effectiveness and to identifying the need and strategies for alternative interventions. The use of a *reflexive journal* (daily record of activities, decisions and rationale, and personal reflections) by the participating professionals is consistent with a reflective approach to practice. *Referential adequacy* (archived, unanalyzed data for future reference) may be easily accomplished when an abundance of data is collected, especially if researchers–evaluators find it feasible to sample from, rather than use all, the available data.

SUMMARY AND CONCLUSIONS

The PCSIM combines ethnographic research methods with PAR, PCSC, and an ecological perspective to transform traditional intervention

TABLE 2.4
Techniques for Ensuring Trustworthiness of Naturalistic Inquiry

Technique	Definition
Prolonged engagement[a]	Investing sufficient time to learn the culture, build trust with stakeholders, understand the scope of target phenomena, and test for misinformation or misinterpretation due to distortion by the researcher or informant
Persistent observation[a]	Continuing process to permit identification and assessment of salient factors, and investigation in sufficient detail to separate "relevant (typical) from irrelevant (atypical)
Triangulation[a]	Data collection, analysis, and interpretation based on multiple sources, methods, investigators, and theories
Peer debriefing[a]	Engage in analytic discussions with neutral peer (e.g., colleague not involved in project)
Member checks[a]	Test veracity of the data, analytic categories (e.g., codes), interpretations, and conclusions with members of stakeholder group, to ensure accurate representation of emic perspective
Thick description[b]	Presentation of procedures, context, and participants in sufficient detail to permit judgment by others of the similarity to potential application sites; specify minimum elements necessary to "re-create" findings
Audit trail[c,d]	Records that include raw data; documentation of all data reduction, analysis, and synthesis process and products; methodological process notes; reflexive notes; and instrument development/piloting techniques
Negative case analysis[a]	Investigate "disconfirming" instance or outlier; continue investigation until all known cases are accounted for, so that data reflect range of variation (vs. normative portrayal)
Reflexive journal[a,b,c,d]	Researcher's personal notes, that is, documentation of researcher's thinking throughout the research process
Referential adequacy[a]	Archiving of a portion of the raw data for subsequent analysis and interpretation, that is, for verification of initial findings and conclusions

Note. See Lincoln and Guba (1985) for detailed discussion of criteria and techniques.
[a] For ensuring credibility (i.e., internal validity). [b] For ensuring transferability (i.e., external validity). [c] For ensuring dependability (i.e., reliability). [d] For ensuring confirmability (i.e., objectivity).

approaches to research-based practice that reflects the cultural experiences and concerns of key stakeholders. Building on PAR methods from applied anthropology and collaborative consultation models from school psychology, we propose a model for engaging stakeholders as partners in the intervention design, implementation, and evaluation. Moreover, we propose the use of ethnographic (qualitative) research methods as tools for data collection throughout the process of program development and evaluation. Ethnographic methods (observation, interview, collecting artifacts) are consistent with data collection methods used by school psychology practitioners and provide a systematic way of addressing ecological factors that are critical to individual functioning. In addition, the use of ethnography helps to ensure that problems and solutions are conceptualized in a culture- or context-specific manner, and thus fosters the translation of evidence-based interventions to real-life settings. In the next three chapters, we describe and illustrate the components of PCSIM (chap. 3, this volume) and its application to creating comprehensive school-based mental health services (chaps. 4 and 5, this volume).

3

COMPONENTS OF THE PARTICIPATORY CULTURE-SPECIFIC INTERVENTION MODEL: AN ILLUSTRATION

In this chapter, we introduce the participatory culture-specific intervention model (PCSIM) as a means for guiding the development of comprehensive school-based mental health services. This model frames the remainder of the book, in which we describe and illustrate the procedures for engaging partners in designing, implementing, and evaluating culture-specific school-based mental health programs. The PCSIM represents an integration of research and intervention that is consistent with current concepts of science-based psychological practice, incorporates characteristics of effective comprehensive programming, and attempts to address the shortcomings of existing models.

The PCSIM is characterized by active participation of key stakeholders in the design, implementation, evaluation, and institutionalization of culture-specific intervention or change efforts such as school-based mental health services. As depicted in Figure 3.1, PCSIM represents an integration of two processes—research and intervention (practice)—that are typically viewed as separate. At the heart of the process is the evolving partnership that is essential to promoting ownership, sustainability, and institutionalization and the continual attention to ecological (culture- and context-specific)

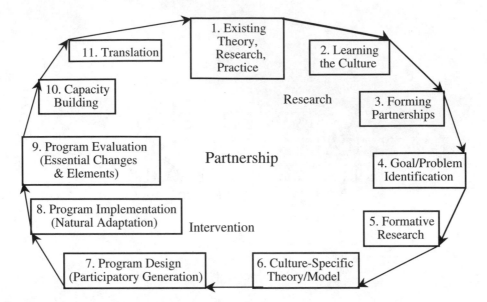

Figure 3.1. Participatory culture-specific intervention model (PCSIM): The model includes 12 components characterized by the integration of 6 research components or phases (1–6), 5 intervention components or phases (7–11), and a central partnership component. The PCSIM is recursive and dynamic and involves the continual exchange between research and intervention. Critical to effective use of PCSIM is the continual reflective application of the research–practice interaction (i.e., research ↔ practice).

fit and program effectiveness. The researchers–interventionists–program developers involve the stakeholders (clients, consultees, representatives of communities or organizations) as partners in the design, implementation, and evaluation of services.

A primary goal of PCSIM is culture specificity through the development of interventions that reflect the shared language, ideas, beliefs, values, and behavioral norms of the members of the target culture (Nastasi, 1998). Thus, understanding the culture of the target population (stakeholders) is considered critical. The development of interventions that are culture specific depends on the use of research methods, such as ethnography, that facilitate understanding of cultural experiences from the perspective of the members or stakeholders. Ethnographic (or other qualitative) research methods are thus integral to formative and evaluative phases of PCSIM. Combined with standardized quantitative methods, they provide the means for understanding the culture of stakeholders and the cultural contributions to mental health of individuals and communities.

EXHIBIT 3.1
Phases of the Participatory Culture-Specific Intervention Model (PCSIM)

Formative (Research) Phases

System Entry

   Phase 1: Existing theory, research, and practice (personal theory)
   Phase 2: Learning the culture
   Phase 3: Forming partnerships

Model Development

   Phase 4: Goal or problem identification
   Phase 5: Formative research
   Phase 6: Culture-specific theory or model

Program (Intervention) Phases

Program Development

   Phase 7: Program design (participatory generation)
   Phase 8: Program implementation (natural adaptation)
   Phase 9: Program evaluation (essential changes and elements)

Program Continuation or Extension

   Phase 10: Capacity building (sustainability and institutionalization)
   Phase 11: Translation (dissemination and deployment)

The 11 phases of PCSIM, listed in Exhibit 3.1, guide program developers through a process that begins with system entry and concludes with program continuation or extension. The formative (research) phases, Phases 1 through 6, include (a) Phases 1 through 3, which collectively represent entry into the system and form the basis for negotiating relationships and program goals; and (b) Phases 4 through 6, which are devoted to development of the theoretical model to guide the articulation of goals and design of the program. The program (intervention) phases, Phases 7 through 11, include (a) Phases 7 through 9, which address the design, implementation, and evaluation of the program; and (b) Phases 10 and 11, which are focused on the continuation or extension of program-related efforts.

Despite the seemingly linear nature of both intervention and research phases, the use of PCSIM requires a recursive approach in which the separate components of intervention and research interact in a dynamic and synergistic manner. Thus, for example, learning the culture not only precedes intervention design but also continues throughout implementation, evaluation, capacity building, and translation. Similarly, learning the culture occurs as researchers examine local theories and practices of stakeholders, form partnerships, conduct formative research, identify the problem, and generate culture-specific theory. The key to recursion is the continual reflective application of the research–practice interaction (i.e., research ↔ practice).

The significance of PCSIM is its potential for facilitating development of socially valid and culturally relevant services, promoting ownership and empowerment among stakeholders who are responsible for sustaining and institutionalizing services, and thereby fostering meaningful and acceptable intervention efforts and sustainable social change (G. L. Anderson, 1989; Meyers & Nastasi, 1998; Nastasi, Varjas, Sarkar, & Jayasena, 1998; Nastasi, Varjas, & Schensul, et al., 2000; J. J. Schensul, 1998). The PCSIM thus provides a mechanism for engaging organizational or community members in developing culture-specific interventions. Furthermore, participatory intervention has the potential for fostering the integration of research and practice, thereby reducing the gap between availability and use of scientifically based interventions.[1] Participatory approaches to intervention and consultation have been used successfully in schools and communities nationally and internationally (e.g., Nastasi et al., 1998–1999; Nastasi, Varjas, Bernstein, & Jayasena, 2000; Nastasi, Varjas, Sarkar, & Jayasena, 1998; Nastasi, Varjas, Schensul, et al., 2000; J. J. Schensul, 1998; J. J. Schensul, 1998–1999).

In the following sections, we describe and illustrate the essential components of PCSIM using an example from our own work. In chapters 4 and 5, the procedures for applying PCSIM to school-based comprehensive mental health services are detailed and illustrated further with school- and community-based applications from our work and that of others.

COMPONENTS OF THE PARTICIPATORY CULTURE-SPECIFIC INTERVENTION MODEL

As depicted in Figure 3.1, the PCSIM is characterized by the integration of 11 complementary research and intervention phases (numbering 6 and 5 phases, respectively), with partnership at its center. These 11 phases and the centralizing partnership constitute the 12 components of PCSIM. In this section, we briefly describe each component. For the sake of clarity, the components are presented in a sequential manner and the phases are artificially separated into research (Phases 1–6) and intervention (Phases 7–11). The participatory culture-specific intervention process, however, is recursive and dynamic. The nonlinear interactive nature of the model is elucidated in the descriptions and illustrations that follow and clarified

---

[1] Several terms have been used to describe interventions whose efficacy or effectiveness is supported by social science or medical research, including *scientifically based*, *science based*, *empirically based*, *evidence based*, *empirically validated*, *empirically supported*, and *supported by outcomes research*.

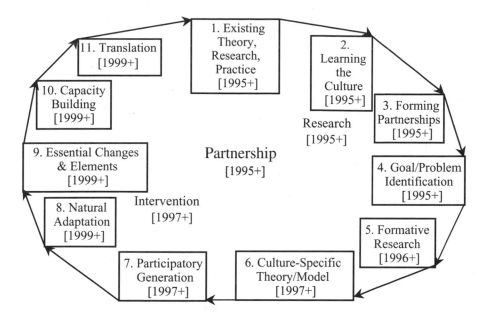

Figure 3.2. Application of the participatory culture-specific intervention model (PCSIM): Sri Lanka Mental Health (SLMH) Project. The SLMH Project reflected the application of the 12 components of PCSIM (see Figure 3.1). Project activities spanned the period from 1995 to 1999. As noted, some activities continue to date.

further through the application of PCSIM to school-based mental health services in chapters 4 and 5.

To illustrate the 12 components of PCSIM, we draw from our work in the Sri Lanka Mental Health (SLMH) Project[2] (Nastasi, Varjas, Bernstein, & Jayasena, 2000; Nastasi, Varjas, Sarkar, & Jayasena, 1998). (See also Nastasi, Varjas, Schensul, et al., 2000, for application of the participatory approach to development of community-based interventions.) The SLMH Project involved the use of PCSIM to conduct formative and intervention research related to the development of school-based mental health services in the urban community of Kandy in the Central Province of Sri Lanka. Figure 3.2 depicts the PCSIM components as they evolved over a period of five years (1995–1999), with extension efforts continuing to date.

[2] Funding for the Sri Lanka Mental Health Project was provided through grants to Bonnie K. Nastasi from the Society for the Study of School Psychology and the University at Albany, State University of New York.

Appendix 3.1 describes timelines, participants, methods, evidence of culture specificity, and outcomes for Phases 1 through 11.

PARTNERSHIP

As depicted in Figures 3.1 and 3.2, partnership is at the center of the PCSIM process. Partners include the researchers–interventionists and representatives of all stakeholder groups that have vested interests or essential resources. In school-based mental health programs, the stakeholders include administrative, teaching, and support staff within the school building or district and other participating agencies (e.g., community mental health, child protection agencies) as well as parents, students, and community leaders and members. Developing a partnership process involves bringing together representatives of all stakeholder groups, establishing an acceptable and effective process for equitable participation, and sustaining communication and participation over time.

The goals of participation are (a) cultural and contextual specificity, (b) sustainability and institutionalization of services, and (c) active involvement, ownership, and empowerment of stakeholders. The expectation is that stakeholders not only are engaged in initial design, implementation, and evaluation of services but also take responsibility for the continuing implementation, monitoring, and revision of services. The capacity for stakeholders to sustain these efforts is dependent on the development of relevant skills. Thus, training in requisite knowledge and skills is an important component of the program development process. Moreover, stakeholders' assumption of ownership for change efforts is dependent on the interventionists' willingness to share control and power. Interventionists must have the capacity to step out of expert roles and engage as equal partners. Establishing and maintaining successful interpersonal relationships are critical to the partnership. Negotiation of partnership is an integral part of the PCSIM process and requires continual monitoring and revisiting throughout the research and intervention phases.

The partners in the SLMH Project included researchers from the United States and Sri Lanka, along with mental health service providers, educators, government administrators, students, and community members from the target community in Sri Lanka. As indicated in the Participants/Informants column of Appendix 3.1, both U.S. and Sri Lankan partners were actively involved in all 11 phases, with representatives of the various stakeholder groups playing different roles throughout the PCSIM process. The active involvement of our Sri Lankan partners was considered essential to the success of the project, particularly to the achievement of culture specificity, and required ongoing attention to the nature and quality of these relationships.

RESEARCH COMPONENTS

The research components of PCSIM are based in participatory action research, as described earlier. The goal of the six research components (Phases 1–6; Figures 3.1 and 3.2) is to develop a culturally and contextually relevant theory that guides the five intervention components (Phases 7–11). Although traditional approaches to intervention are often guided by theory and research, PCSIM requires explicit research activities to ensure an appropriate theoretical–empirical base for the target population and context. In this section, the research components are presented as formal phases that precede intervention design. In reality, the phases are continually revisited during each of the intervention phases (from intervention design to dissemination).

Phase 1: Existing Theory, Research, and Practice (Personal Theory)

Phase 1 constitutes a formal phase devoted to considering personal perspectives (i.e., personal theories)—based on relevant theory, research, and applied experiences—that guide the work and actions of researchers–interventionists and key stakeholders. The explicit focus on personal theories reflects recognition of the potential influence of each individual's views and experiences on the participatory process and effectiveness of change efforts. Successful articulation and communication of personal theories are likely to be influenced by efforts to learn about the cultures represented by stakeholders.

In the SLMH Project, we used a conceptual model of mental health, based in psychology and anthropology, as the starting point for engaging in the PCSIM process (see Figure 3.3; Nastasi & DeZolt, 1994; Nastasi et al., 1998–1999; Nastasi, Varjas, Sarkar, & Jayasena, 1998). This model depicts the synergistic relationship between individual and cultural factors that influence psychological functioning and mental health. Individual (or personal) factors include culturally valued competencies (e.g., personal strength, sense of humor, musical ability), personal resources (e.g., coping skills, self-efficacy, interpersonal skills), and personal vulnerability (e.g., family history of mental illness, personal history of school adjustment problems). Cultural factors include cultural norms (e.g., regarding gender roles or relationships), social–cultural stressors (e.g., poverty, family conflict, school violence), social–cultural resources (e.g., teachers, family members, school psychologist), socialization practices (e.g., discipline strategies, instruction),

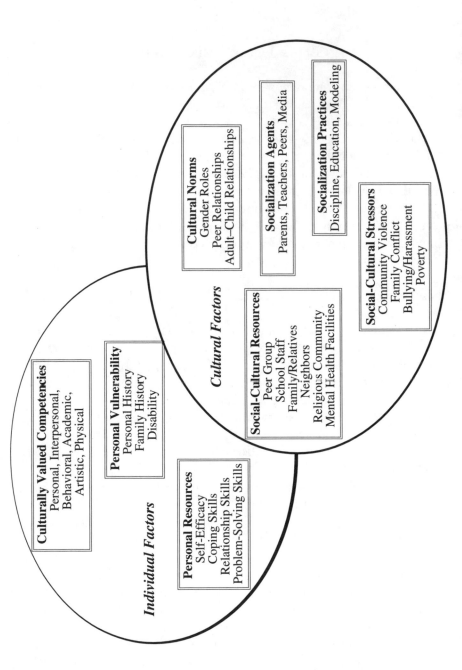

Figure 3.3. Conceptual model of mental health: This model guided formative research that culminated in the development of a culture-specific mental health conceptual model (depicted in Figure 3.4), intervention program, and evaluation tools. From "Participatory Model of Mental Health Programming: Lessons Learned From Work in a Developing Country," by B. K. Nastasi, K. Varjas, S. Sarkar, and A. Jayasena, 1998, *School Psychology Review, 27,* p. 265. Copyright 1998 by the National Association of School Psychologists. Adapted with permission.

and socialization agents (e.g., adults, peers, media). Current mental health status is considered to reflect the interaction of these individual and cultural factors. In the SLMH Project, this conceptual model provided the basis for engaging in dialogue with partners, learning the culture, identifying mental health goals, collecting formative data, and formulating culture-specific theory.

Phase 2: Learning the Culture

Phase 2 involves efforts to understand the cultural experiences, language, beliefs, values, and norms of the various stakeholder groups. The initiation of "learning the culture" typically coincides with efforts by researchers–interventionists to gain entry into the target system (e.g., school, community). During this phase, efforts are made to identify *cultural brokers* who are members of the culture and facilitate acceptance into and interpretation of the culture. The goal of this phase is consistent with the goal of ethnography, that is, to gain knowledge of the culture from the perspective of its members. Ethnographic research methods are critical to implementation of this phase, as illustrated in chapter 4. As noted earlier, the process of learning the culture continues beyond this initial entry. As researchers–interventionists begin to learn the culture, they also begin the process of forming partnerships.

In the SLMH Project, learning the culture involved the use of several ethnographic methods: participant observation, key-informant interviews, collection of artifacts such as local newspapers and popular mental health literature, and use of secondary data from a project on sexual risk (Appendix 3.1). These data were critical to assessing cultural definitions of mental health, perceptions of need across the various stakeholder groups, available and potential formal and informal resources for mental health service delivery, and interest in school-based mental health. In addition to contributing to the formative research process, the study of culture was important for identifying potential partners for conducting research and intervention.

Phase 3: Forming Partnerships

Phase 3 interventionists–researchers begin to establish relationships with and among stakeholders, thus initiating the interpersonal participatory process that continues throughout and beyond the formal intervention project. The process of negotiating relationships with and among partners is ongoing, with initiation of new relationships and renegotiation of existing relationships continuing as the partners enter subsequent phases of the process.

Critical to active participation and culture specificity is the involvement of cultural brokers, defined as

> individuals who can effectively bridge the gap between our cultural experiences and those of the population we serve. The cultural broker has access to and acceptability in the target culture or context, has expert status in the culture, can facilitate entry into the culture or system, and can interpret experiences from the perspective of the members of the culture. In a sense, a cultural broker is similar to a translator or interpreter in terms of being able to facilitate communication between individuals who speak different languages. The role of the cultural broker, however, extends beyond that of the translator/interpreter of the language and serves instead as an interpreter/expert of the culture and a liaison between the researcher/consultant and the researched/consultees. Whereas the translator may be viewed as a tool for facilitating communication, the cultural broker is viewed as a consulting partner. (Nastasi, Varjas, Bernstein, & Jayasena, 2000, pp. 405, 407)

In the SLMH Project, partnerships grew out of previously established relationships between social science and medical professionals (dating back a decade) and ongoing work on a sexual risk project in the target community. Specific attention to partnership formation for the SLMH Project, however, began during two visits to Sri Lanka (Appendix 3.1). The initial partnerships with Sri Lankan researchers were extended to include professionals and lay members of the educational and mental health (or social service) communities at national, provincial, city, and neighborhood levels. Through the use of ethnographic methods (e.g., key-informant and in-depth interviews), seminars, and meetings, we identified potential partners and explored their concerns and interests related to the mental health of children and adolescents. One of our professional partners (Asoka Jayasena, University of Peradeniya) became a key collaborator and cultural broker. Jayasena, an educational sociologist and teacher educator, was extremely knowledgeable about the educational system in Sri Lanka and was highly respected by national, provincial, and local administrators and educators. She participated actively in all project activities. She initiated contacts with educational agencies, co-conducted interviews (conducted in two languages), participated in data analysis and interpretation, and collaborated in development and implementation of the intervention. Most important, she served as a "cultural interpreter," assisting the U.S. researchers in understanding cultural concepts and the meaning of language and actions of other participants. A second cultural broker in the project was an individual hired to translate materials produced by students during the intervention. This individual not only did direct translation of student work to English but also met with the U.S. researchers on a regular basis to share his cultural interpretation of situations depicted by students.

Phase 4: Goal or Problem Identification

During Phase 4, partners initially identify the target concern or problem and the desired goal or outcome that will become the focus of their collaborative efforts. In some cases, the stakeholders have identified a general goal or concern that led to enlisting the expertise of the interventionists. In other cases, the target goal or problem is identified by researchers or interventionists who are external or internal to the organization. In either instance, it behooves program planners to engage stakeholders in specifying the goal or problem so that it becomes ecologically valid and realistically achievable or solvable. It is not uncommon for initial foci to mask underlying issues that are not visible or are difficult to articulate. For this reason, the definition and elaboration of goals or concerns require data collection about the individual and ecological factors that influence and surround the target issue.

In the SLMH Project, the identification of short- and long-term goals reflected the culmination of work conducted during Phases 1 through 3. As depicted in Appendix 3.1, the data collected during system entry activities helped to establish the needs for mental health services and led to the formulation of goals related to mental health service delivery. These goals then guided subsequent formative research and culture-specific model development.

Phase 5: Formative Research

In this formative research phase (Phase 5), the partners (researchers–interventionists and stakeholders) gather data about the target goal or problem to fully articulate the factors that influence the desired outcome or target problem and to establish goals for the intervention. Moreover, formative research influences the generation of culture-specific or local theory that guides intervention design. Data are collected and analyzed using ethnographic research methods (e.g., observation, interview, survey). The participatory nature of PCSIM requires that stakeholders are involved in data collection, analysis, and interpretation. Their successful involvement depends on development of research skills and the capacity of the researchers–interventionists to provide necessary training. Equipping community members with research skills is considered fundamental to empowerment and institutionalization as well as to the generation of interventions that reflect local culture, resources, and needs.

The conceptual model identified in Phase 1 of the SLMH Project (see Figure 3.3) was the foundation for formative research in an urban community of Sri Lanka that culminated in the development of a culture-specific mental health promotion program and culture-specific assessment tools for program evaluation (Nastasi, Varjas, Bernstein, & Jayasena, 2000; Nastasi, Varjas, Sarkar, & Jayasena, 1998). We used ethnographic methods—observations, in-depth interviews, focus group interviews, and collection of artifacts—to gather data about relevant individual and cultural factors from students, teachers, and administrators in 18 schools (see Appendix 3.1). Data were collected, analyzed, and interpreted by the team of U.S. and Sri Lankan researchers.

Phase 6: Culture-Specific (Local) Theory or Model

Researchers–interventionists and stakeholders use formative research data, in conjunction with existing theory and research, to generate culture-specific hypotheses and recommendations for action. Their task is to identify the factors that seem to influence the target goal or problem and thus are likely targets for intervention. The outcome of Phase 6 is articulation of a model for explaining the target phenomena (e.g., school violence) based on individual and social–cultural factors within the target context. The resultant local theory guides the intervention or practice phases of PCSIM.

Interpretation of formative research data from the SLMH Project led to the development of a culture-specific model of mental health and a five-year plan for securing funding and initiating intervention efforts. The culture-specific model of mental health, depicted in Figure 3.4 (Varjas, 2003), is a modification of the initial conceptual model (Figure 3.3) and portrays the interaction of individual characteristics with cultural factors from four key ecological contexts (family, school, peer group, and community). This model guided the development of assessment–evaluation tools and an intervention program.

INTERVENTION (PRACTICE) COMPONENTS

The five intervention components are an extension and redefinition of traditional steps of intervention—design, implementation, and evaluation. During these five phases (Phases 7–11; see Figure 3.1 and Exhibit 3.1), interventionists–researchers engage stakeholders in planning, carrying out, evaluating, institutionalizing, and disseminating an intervention that is based in the formative research and culture-specific theory generated in earlier formal research phases. The partners may choose to select or modify existing interventions and evaluation tools or develop new procedures specific to the needs and resources of the target context. Successful participation depends on the skills of stakeholders and capacity of researchers–interventionists to provide necessary training. It is possible that additional

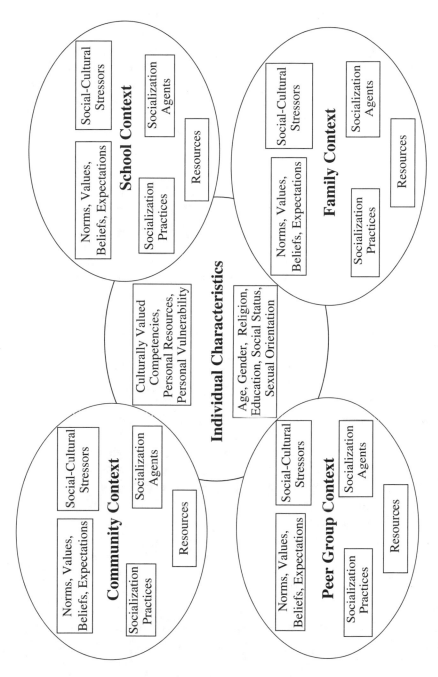

Figure 3.4. Culture-specific model of mental health: Sri Lanka Mental Health (SLMH) Project. This culture-specific model is a modification of the initial conceptual model (Figure 3.3) and reflects the interaction of individual factors with cultural factors from four key ecological contexts: school, family, peer group, and community. This model was the basis for developing an intervention program and assessment/evaluation tools. From *A Participatory Culture-Specific Consultation (PCSC) Approach to Intervention Development*, by K. M. Varjas, 2003, p. 164. Unpublished doctoral dissertation, University at Albany, State University of New York. Adapted with permission of the author.

stakeholders with expertise in the selected intervention and evaluation procedures become involved during these phases.

The following component descriptions are presented in a step-by-step manner. In reality, generation (design), adaptation (implementation), evaluation, capacity building, and dissemination are ongoing and interactive. For example, capacity building requires reconsideration of program design; evaluation is critical to the adaptation of the design during implementation; and the capacity for translating the intervention to other contexts requires evaluation of both program implementation and outcomes.

Phase 7: Program Design (Participatory Generation)

The process of intervention design in PCSIM is best described as participatory generation. During Phase 7, researchers–interventionists work together with stakeholders to create or socially construct interventions (e.g., Serrano-Garcia, 1990, described the process as the social construction of interventions). Consistent with the initial design stage of traditional intervention approaches, participatory generation involves decision making about program goals and specific features of the intervention (e.g., curriculum content, intervention techniques, staffing). In this generation process, partners use data from formative research to (a) identify and describe individual and cultural variables related to the target outcomes, (b) generate local theory, (c) identify culture- or context-specific goals and intervention strategies, and (d) design a culture or context-specific intervention. Thus, the program design process extends the work of Phases 1 through 6. Negotiating the multiple perspectives of different stakeholders is critical to the social construction of the intervention and requires effective methods for communication and consensus building (articulated in chap. 5, this volume). Furthermore, the generation process requires that partners continue to engage in a reflective process of examining personal theory, learning the culture, establishing and maintaining interpersonal relationships, collecting data, and revising local theory as they work to devise an intervention plan.

In the SLMH Project, Phase 7 activities involved the development of culture-specific assessment tools (e.g., student self-report measures of sense of competence, perceived culturally valued competencies, stressors, social supports, and coping strategies; discussed further in chap. 5, this volume), a mental health promotion curriculum, and teacher training materials.[3] The mental health curriculum, designed to be implemented by teachers, reflected the culture-specific model of mental health depicted in Figure 3.4. For

---

[3] Additional information and copies of intervention, training, and assessment tools can be obtained from Bonnie K. Nastasi.

example, the objectives of the program included the following: (a) identifying and strengthening socially valued competencies, (b) identifying stressors and resources across the key ecological contexts, (c) considering feelings as signals of stress, (d) enhancing coping skills, and (e) minimizing stress through use of coping skills, including accessing available social supports. In addition, the curriculum was structured so that students had the opportunity to explore individually and with peers (in small groups) the key people, expectations, stressors, resources, and coping strategies relevant to adaptation in each ecological context. Furthermore, the sequence of the curriculum reflected the relative cultural emphasis on the larger collective (i.e., community) and smaller social contexts (family and peer). Consistent with values reflected in formative data, the curriculum focused on the individual in relationship to others. To facilitate this depiction of self in relationship to others, students constructed ecomaps (visual depictions of self and significant others and the nature of those relationships as stressful or supportive; Compton & Galaway, 1989) for each ecological context.

Phase 8: Program Implementation (Natural Adaptation)

Within PCSIM, the concept of natural adaptation reflects the focus on modification of the planned intervention to meet the needs and resources within the specific intervention context, in contrast to strict adherence to the plan during implementation in traditional intervention models. The assumption is that an intervention based on formative research with the target population cannot account for all individual and contextual variations (e.g., if one were to implement across several classrooms). The goal of natural adaptation (Phase 8) is to make adjustments to ensure optimal fit of the intervention with context and recipients (i.e., to achieve an ecological niche as defined by Bronfenbrenner, 1989) while retaining the core aspects of the intervention (i.e., maintaining intervention integrity).[4] Consistent with the participatory process, adaptations are negotiated with stakeholders.

In-depth documentation (part of the evaluation component) during implementation serves multiple purposes. It permits monitoring of unplanned modifications, provides data to support planned modifications, and facilitates the identification of critical elements (those essential to achieving program outcomes) and noncritical elements (those that necessarily vary to achieve the optimal fit but do not interfere with program effectiveness). The iterative action research process within the phase of natural adaptation guides documentation and planned modification.

---

[4]*Natural adaptation* is consistent with the concepts of mutual adaptation (McLaughlin, 1976, 1990), proadaptation (Weissberg, 1990), and reinvention (Blakely et al., 1987).

The rationale for adaptation is that modifications are necessary to accommodate variations in recipients, program implementers, and settings and to ensure sustainability. The necessity of modifications for ensuring successful program implementation is supported by research on organizational change and social program innovations (McLaughlin, 1976, 1990). Given the potential variation with broad-scale application of an intervention (e.g., system, community, nationwide, global), it is critical that the adaptation process (and its documentation) occurs each time the program is implemented in a new setting or with new participants (implementers or recipients). The failure to address adaptation issues may contribute to difficulties in transferring interventions across contexts or participants (i.e., to translation or deployment).

In the SLMH Project, program implementation involved teacher training and delivery of the curriculum in an after-school program (see Appendix 3.1). A process of on-site consultation with teachers and monitoring of curriculum delivery resulted in modifications of the intervention process and content to meet the needs of program participants. For example, in response to teachers' requests, abbreviated teacher curriculum guides were developed to facilitate ease of use, and graphic time indicators were added to signal transitions from one activity to another. Sri Lankan and U.S. interventionists–researchers participated collaboratively in the consultation, monitoring, and adaptation processes. For example, the researchers worked in cross-cultural teams while on-site, to facilitate translation, cultural interpretation, and participatory problem solving with teachers.

Phase 9: Program Evaluation (Essential Changes and Elements)

Phase 9, the phase of essential changes parallels the evaluation stage of traditional intervention and integrates the evaluation of process and outcomes into a continual seamless process. Although the primary focus is typically the effectiveness (or outcome) of the intervention, in this model critical attention is given also to intervention acceptability, social validity, and integrity and how these factors interact to influence outcomes. Furthermore, the focus on outcomes extends beyond immediate intended effects to unintended outcomes, long-term outcomes, and sustainability and institutionalization of intervention efforts. Assessment of essential changes (i.e., progress toward program goals) occurs at multiple points during and after the intervention. To determine if adequate progress is being made, performance at any point in time is compared with the desired competence level or program outcome. The concept of essential changes thus reflects the notion of sufficient movement in the direction of intervention goals. Follow-up evaluation focuses on issues of maintenance of program effects as well as sustainability and institutionalization of program efforts. In addition, essential changes are linked to documented components of the intervention to determine which are essential to achieving outcomes (i.e., to identify critical elements). Furthermore, evaluation data are used to inform subsequent practice as well as extant theory and research, thus completing the action research and PCSIM cycle.

Evaluation of the SLMH intervention program involved the use of several ethnographic techniques (see Appendix 3.1) by on-site researchers. Evaluation activities were conducted throughout program implementation to monitor acceptability, social validity, integrity, and impact and to facilitate adaptation to the needs of participating teachers and students. For example, observation of intervention sessions, formal and informal dialogue with teachers, and collection of student products were essential to monitoring progress toward program goals and determining needed modifications. Culture-specific pre–post measures (developed from formative research data) were administered to the program participants and randomly assigned control participants to examine program effectiveness. (Examples of these evaluation tools can be found in chap. 5, this volume.)

Phase 10: Capacity Building (Sustainability and Institutionalization)

In this phase of intervention, program developers collaborate with stakeholders in planning and implementing strategies to ensure that change efforts become an integral part of the organization or institution. One goal is to foster sustainability of change efforts by creating an infrastructure that supports continued intervention activities, that is, institutionalizing newly adopted programs. Institutionalization requires the availability of necessary resources, including professional expertise, staff, administrative structure, equipment, supplies, and funding. In addition, ensuring continued change efforts requires a mechanism for staff development, monitoring and evaluation, and adaptation of programs to meeting changing cultural, contextual, and individual needs.

A broader goal of capacity building is to enable the organization and its stakeholders to engage in continued efforts to address self-identified challenges or crises and to foster successful functioning and well-being as they deem appropriate. This goal is consistent with the definition of capacity building as person-centered development, that is, as a process for adaptation that focuses on strengthening the capability of individuals within an institution or society to achieve objectives they identify and define (Eade, 1997). Thus, the goal is ensuring human and organizational capacity relevant not only to the immediate project but also to long-term development. This more general capacity is dependent on the development of human resources and organizational infrastructure necessary for engaging in the PCSIM process independent of the expert program developers, interventionists, researchers, or consultants who facilitated the initial project. This approach is inconsistent with current practices in program or project development and funding, which are typically limited to design, implementation, and evaluation of a specific time-limited project. The relatively short-term nature (e.g., 3 to 5 years) of these projects impedes the establishment of long-term capacity. Furthermore, traditional project-specific work seldom addresses capacity building as a primary goal.

Although we identify this as one of the final phases in PCSIM, capacity building begins in the initial stages (e.g., with examining personal theory, forming partnerships, learning the culture) and continues throughout the PCSIM process (e.g., during design, implementation, and evaluation). Efforts to foster ownership by and empowerment of stakeholders, both critical to program success and capacity building, begin early on. In addition, activities devoted to staff development in research, intervention, and evaluation also help to build organizational capacity. Finally, as partners move toward completion of formal program efforts, program planners gradually withdraw their direct involvement and provide indirect support through consultation. Follow-up support continues indefinitely, although the successful consultants (program developers) work to foster independent functioning of stakeholders and eventual termination of their role within a given project. Thus, success is marked by the willingness of the system to assume both responsibility and credit for the success or failure of not only project-specific efforts but also more global and enduring change or development efforts.

As reflected in Appendix 3.1, capacity-building activities in the SLMH Project included disseminating findings to the participating school staff and local researchers and educators, preparing Sri Lankan researchers and teachers-in-training in the research and intervention methods, and providing culture-specific intervention and evaluation tools for use in Sri Lankan schools. Consistent with PCSIM, the capacity-building activities began in the early phases of the project (e.g., training graduate students in Sri Lanka in ethnographic methods) and continue to date through ongoing collaboration with Asoka Jayasena.

Phase 11: Translation (Dissemination and Deployment)

This final phase, Phase 11, is consistent with traditional efforts to disseminate findings of projects to stakeholders and other lay and professional audiences but goes beyond these efforts in several ways. First, activities of this phase are devoted to formalizing the program planners' reflections on practice related to the intervention. That is, the individual interventionist–researcher is expected to examine the knowledge gained through participation in the project and consider implications for personal theory that guides practice in general. Second, the interventionist–researcher can guide the reflective process for other stakeholders, as a concluding activity of the project, thus fostering reflective practice as a component of capacity building. Third, the interventionist can assist stakeholders in other contexts in translating their evidence-based practice through replication of the PCSIM process. This notion of translation is consistent with the concept of deployment as a process of applying evidence-based interventions in real-life or field contexts coupled with research on the necessary conditions for successful application (NIMH, 2001a).

Deployment research is focused on studying the process and outcome of a previously validated intervention and the factors that influence the acceptability, integrity, and effectiveness in natural (field, real-life) settings, and it requires input of stakeholders who are expected to provide and receive intervention services. The National Advisory Mental Health Council Workgroup on Child and Adolescent Mental Health Intervention Development and Deployment, sponsored by the National Institute of Mental Health, called for systematic attention to intervention deployment and use of a cyclical process that ensures feedback from deployment research to other forms of basic and intervention research (i.e., development, testing, and synthesis) that precede deployment efforts (NIMH, 2001a). We propose that PCSIM provides the mechanism not only for conducting deployment research but also for integrating deployment questions into all phases of the basic research to deployment cycle.

In the SLMH Project (see Appendix 3.1), reflection by researchers–interventionists and participating teachers was facilitated through a series of discussion sessions immediately following the conclusion of the intervention. Discussion was focused on lessons learned, application of techniques to classroom and school contexts, and implications for theory, research, and practice. Dissemination activities were extended beyond the local context (described in Phase 10) to professional audiences in Sri Lanka, the United States, India, and internationally through presentations and publications. Finally, translation efforts are ongoing as we negotiate extended work in Sri Lanka, India, and the United States through application of PCSIM to develop school- and community-based mental health programs.

SUMMARY

The PCSIM provides a formalized process for the development of comprehensive mental health services that target both individual and social–cultural change. The model extends the key components of existing models for comprehensive service provision (see Exhibit 1.2 in chap. 1, this volume) as it

- promotes not only evidence-based practice but also the continual integration of research and practice in a reflective, participatory, and interdisciplinary manner;
- uses cultural brokers to facilitate communication between researchers–interventionists and consumers;
- explicitly focuses on ecological factors at local and societal levels;
- provides a mechanism for the sustained and meaningful involvement of stakeholders in decision making and change efforts through the development of relevant skills;
- capitalizes on emerging cultural issues and changes as focal points for intervention;
- is aimed at both individualized and institutionalized change with a primary focus on capacity building; and
- is a means for conducting intervention research in a way that addresses questions of deployment and translation throughout the research process rather than as a separate process.

Application of the Participatory Culture-Specific Intervention Model (PCSIM):
Sri Lanka Mental Health (SLMH) Project

Phase	Timeline	Participants/informants	Methods	Culture specificity	Outcomes
Phase 1: Existing theory, research, and practice	1995–1999	Sri Lanka: educational sociologist–teacher educator, local psychiatrists, teachers, students, school administrators, provincial office of education director and staff, university faculty and students, community members United States: school psychologist–researcher and graduate students	Participant observation, key-informant interviews, in-depth individual and group interviews, artifacts, meetings, participatory workshop and seminars, self-reflection and dialogue	Culture-specific identification and definition of individual and cultural constructs relevant to mental health, consistent with the guiding conceptual model, and informed by formative research and interactions with stakeholders (Nastasi, Varjas, Sarkar, & Jayasena, 1998)	Identified conceptual model of mental health to guide initial work; modified the model on the basis of formative research and dialogue with Sri Lankan stakeholders
Phase 2: Learning the culture	1995–1996 (2 visits; 3 months)	Sri Lanka: psychiatrists, teachers, teachers in training, teacher educators, community members, sociologists, anthropologists, director of nongovernmental organization addressing women's issues United States: school psychologist–researcher, medical and educational anthropologists	Participant observation in schools, community, university, tuition institution, teacher training college; key-informant interviews; artifacts—local newspaper; social science literature on history, social customs, traditions, language, culture-specific fiction, popular mental health literature; secondary data analysis (project on sexual risk)	Suicide rate second highest in the world, highly publicized and sensationalized in local newspaper (e.g., drama of lost love), high rate of completion due to method (ingesting readily available insecticide); students have high anxiety about academic achievement; family problems (and major women's concerns) include alcoholism, domestic abuse, poverty; teachers ill-prepared to deal with learning and behavioral problems; few psychiatrists and no psychologists in country; no psychological services in schools; large school and classroom population; teacher–student ratio is 1 to 50; unsuccessful efforts in past to prepare teachers as counselors	Identified need for and interest (at all levels of the system) in school-based mental health services, teacher preparation regarding mental health, preparation of mental health personnel

(continued)

Phase	Timeline	Participants/informants	Methods	Culture specificity	Outcomes
Phase 3: Forming partnerships	1996–1997 (2 visits; 3 months)	Sri Lanka: educational sociologist–teacher educator; local psychiatrists; representative of national ministry of education; provincial office of education director and staff; local schools—principals, teachers, students; university faculty and students; community members/parents United States: school psychologist–researcher and doctoral student–research assistant	Key-informant interviews; in-depth individual and group interviews; participatory seminar of representatives from stakeholder groups; contact and meetings with individuals from all levels of the system	Weak or nonexistent links between education and mental health community; shared interests in school-based mental health services; interest and commitment at community, school, university, provincial, and national levels in developing school-based mental health services	Forming of partnerships with key stakeholders at local–provincial levels
Phase 4: Goal/problem identification	1995–1997 (see above)	All of the above	All of the above	Lack of accessible mental health services for children and adolescents; need for school-based mental health services, ranging from prevention to treatment; need for mental health personnel and teacher preparation in mental health issues	Formulation of long- and short-term goals related to development of school-based mental health services in the country, with initial efforts in Central Province; efforts to seek funding at national and international levels
Phase 5: Formative research	1996–1997	Sri Lanka: educational sociologist, educational research assistants, provincial director of education, 18 Central Province schools—principals, teachers, students, parents United States: school psychologist–researcher and doctoral students–research assistants	Observations in schools and classrooms, in-depth semistructured individual and focus group interviews, artifacts (e.g., posted notices, school rules, discipline records and policies)	Culture-specific definitions of individual and cultural constructs relevant to mental health—specifically, personal resources, personal vulnerability, culturally valued competencies, social–cultural stressors, cultural norms, socialization practices, social–cultural resources (Nastasi, Varjas, Sarkar, & Jayasena, 1998)	Culture-specific model for mental health promotion, representing the integration of existing theory and research with the formative research data (thus combining etic and emic perspectives, respectively)

| Phase 6: Culture-specific theory/model | 1997–1998 (2 visits, 3 months) | Sri Lanka: educational sociologist; psychiatrist; university and teacher training college faculty; university social science, medical, and educational researchers; provincial education ministry agents; university students in social sciences and education; community members United States: school psychologist–researcher | Participatory workshop and seminars for stakeholders in Central Province to disseminate findings and proposed culture-specific model and gather interpretations, hypotheses, and implications/recommendations for future action | Recommendations focused on culture-specific issues: decreasing teacher–student ratios; providing mental health education for teachers and parents; addressing gender issues in school practices/norms; promoting school–parent–community partnerships; reducing academic pressure; promoting collaboration among youth service organizations; revising educational and teacher training practices; preparing mental health service providers (e.g., school psychologists); and developing school-based mental health services (Nastasi, Varjas, Sarkar, & Jayasena, 1998) | Development of five-year plan for school-based mental health promotion in Sri Lanka, with the following objectives: professional preparation of teachers and mental health service providers; development of mental health promotion curriculum for schools; program development and evaluation research; establish infrastructure for comprehensive mental health service delivery for school-age population to seek funding at national and international levels; participation of U.S. psychologist and Sri Lankan psychiatrist in WHO seminar on school-based mental health promotion efforts, with funding from U.S. university and UNICEF; secured funding for research to develop and test culture-specific assessment tools and school-based mental health promotion intervention, from Society for the Study of School Psychology |

(continued)

Phase	Timeline	Participants/informants	Methods	Culture specificity	Outcomes
Phase 7: Program design (participatory generation)	1997–1998 (see above); 1999 (1 visit; 3 months)	Sri Lanka: educational sociologist–teacher educator, university education faculty and students, provincial director of education, school principal, teachers, and students. United States: school psychologist–researcher; doctoral students in school and educational psychology	Develop student and teacher questionnaires; develop intervention process and content (curriculum); develop teacher training process and content. Translate all materials to primary language of Sinhala; select schools and secure permission for pilot of questionnaire and intervention program from provincial director of education and principals of participating schools; pilot and revise assessment tools	Content of assessment tools, intervention curriculum, and teacher training reflected culture-specific definitions of key constructs (based on formative research described above) and primary language; development of intervention program to be implemented by teachers and teachers in training, capitalizing on existing resources	Culture-specific assessment tools, mental health promotion curriculum, and teacher training materials
Phase 8: Program implementation (natural adaptation)	1999	Sri Lanka: educational sociologist–teacher educator, educational research assistants–consultants, university education students as teaching assistants, school principal, teachers, and students. United States: school psychologist–researcher; doctoral students in school psychology as research assistants/consultants	Teacher training using collaborative consultation model; implementation of teacher training and intervention in one school, using experimental, pre–post design to test acceptability, integrity, and efficacy; collaboration of Sri Lanka and U.S. research–consultant teams; participatory process of monitoring and adapting program to culture and context	Use of culture-specific (and language-specific) teacher training materials and intervention curriculum; implementation of the intervention (i.e., front-line work) by members of the culture; collaboration of on-site researchers and consultants from Sri Lanka and the United States in teacher training and intervention	Adaptation of intervention, assessment, and training materials developed in Phase 7, to meet the needs of participants—school administrators, teachers, students, intervention staff
Phase 9: Program evaluation (essential changes and elements)	1999	Sri Lanka: educational sociologist–teacher educator, educational research assistants, university education students as teaching assistants, school principal, teachers, and students. United States: school psychologist–researcher; doctoral students in school psychology as research assistants/consultants	Process and outcome evaluation, using ethnographic techniques: observation, interviews, logs, journals, culture-specific pre–post questionnaire, acceptability questionnaire, curriculum-based assessment, session notes, and other artifacts	Use of culture- and language-specific evaluation materials; integration of evaluation tools into curriculum and consultation activities; implementation of evaluation methods (i.e., front-line work) by members of the culture; collaboration of on-site researchers and consultants from Sri Lanka and the United States	Documentation of session-by-session progress of teachers and students toward program goals; evidence of impact based on culture-specific assessment tools; monitoring and documentation of acceptability to teachers, students, administrator, intervention staff

Phase 10: Capacity building (sustainability and institutionalization)	1999+ (ongoing/ planned)	Sri Lanka: educational sociologist–teacher educator, educational research assistants, university education students as teaching assistants, school principal, teachers, and students	Dissemination of results and materials to professional and educational community in Sri Lanka	[Ongoing activities] Development of expertise and identification of resources within the existing culture
		United States: school psychologist–researcher, doctoral students in school psychology as research assistants–consultants	Preparation of researchers, consultants, and teaching staff in skills necessary to continue the work	Empowerment and ownership by individuals and institutions at multiple levels within the culture (e.g., local, provincial, national) who can continue teacher preparation and program research, development and evaluation activities
			Ongoing consultation with Sri Lankan stakeholders, with periodic visits from U.S. consultants	
			Sabbatical of educational sociologist–teacher educator in the United States to work with U.S. school psychologist–researcher	
			Extension of program implementation to other schools and provinces; development of related projects to extend focus of mental health programs (e.g., school-based sexual-risk prevention programs)	
			Seeking funds to continue SLMH and to pursue extensions	

(continued)

Phase	Timeline	Participants/informants	Methods	Culture specificity	Outcomes
Phase 11: Translation (dissemination and deployment)	1999+ (ongoing/planned)	Sri Lanka: educational sociologist–teacher educator, educational research assistants, university education students as teaching assistants, school principal, teachers, and students United States: school psychologist–researcher, doctoral students in school psychology as research assistants–consultants, health and mental health professionals and social science researchers as new partners for deployment of model in U.S. communities with Southeast Asian populations India: social science researchers and mental health professionals as new partners for deployment of model in urban communities in India	Dissemination of results and materials to professional and educational communities in Sri Lanka, India, the United States, and internationally through conferences, publications, and local presentations Establishing new partnerships and negotiating "contracts" for deployment research in new contexts with Asian populations (United States and India), which will culminate in replication of PCSIM process	Dissemination includes information about SLMH program and use of PCSIM to replicate process to ensure culture specificity Negotiations of deployment activities include strategies for studying local culture and developing or adapting the conceptual model and intervention to meet culture-specific needs and resources Replication of PCSIM process in each new context	[Ongoing activities]

Note. For more detailed information about the Sri Lanka Mental Health Project, see Nastasi; Varjas; Varjas, Bernstein, and Jayasena (2000) and Nastasi, Varjas, Sarkar, and Jayasena (1998). Additional information can be obtained from Bonnie K. Nastasi. WHO = World Health Organization; UNICEF = United Nations Children's Fund.

4

PARTICIPATORY CULTURE-SPECIFIC INTERVENTION: FORMATIVE (RESEARCH) PHASES

In the next two chapters, the procedures for the application of the participatory culture-specific intervention model (PCSIM) to school-based mental health programs are detailed. These chapters are designed to guide program planners (interventionists, researchers), working in partnership with stakeholders,[1] in the use of PCSIM to create comprehensive school-based mental health services that meet the criteria outlined in Exhibit 1.2 (chap. 1, this volume; see also Nastasi, 1998, 2000). In this chapter we

---

[1] The term *program planners* refers to applied researchers and interventionists who have the responsibility of working in partnership with stakeholders and guiding the process of program planning, implementation, and evaluation. Examples of program planners include psychologists, mental health professionals, medical personnel, university faculty, and researchers or interventionists from community-based organizations or government agencies. They may be employed within the school district or contracted as external agents. The term *stakeholders* refers to those parties with vested interests or necessary resources who work in partnership with program planners and are expected to assume ownership and responsibility for sustaining and institutionalizing program efforts. Stakeholders relevant to comprehensive school-based mental health programming include students, parents, teachers, school administrators, school-based mental health and other support staff, community members, political leaders, and administrators and staff from community-based medical, mental health, social service, or other organizations that represent community interests. The term *partners* is used to refer collectively to the program planners and stakeholders who are involved in any given project.

describe and illustrate procedures relevant to the formative (research) phases, Phases 1 through 6 (see Exhibit 3.1 and Figure 3.1, chap. 3, this volume).

To facilitate application of PCSIM, we outline in tabular form the key considerations for each phase, including focus, participants, strategies or methods, tasks and activities, requisite skills, and challenges and opportunities. In addition, we provide tools such as lists of questions to guide planning and data collection, checklists for monitoring, and references to practical guides and other resource materials. In the context of program phases, we describe methods for conducting action research, participatory consultation, and ethnography. We also provide examples from our work and the work of other researchers and practitioners to illustrate phase activities. Finally, we discuss challenges and issues that confront program planners within respective phases.

An underlying assumption of the PCSIM is that no one program, despite prior empirical validation, can meet the needs of all individuals or contexts, thus necessitating the use of a participatory action research process for each application. When minimal or no information is available, the process must be comprehensive and in-depth. When one is attempting to translate or transfer an evidenced-based program to similar populations and settings, a streamlined version of the process can be used. Nevertheless, the essential features of participation and reflective practice are necessary in all instances. Thus, it is critical that stakeholders are involved in the process of planning, implementing, and evaluating and that decision making is linked to data specific to the target population and context.

The scope of comprehensive school-based mental health programming necessitates collaboration among mental health professionals and other stakeholders. Although we acknowledge that partners play varying roles and bring a range of skills to the process, we approach our discussion from the perspective of the mental health professional (program planner) responsible for facilitating the participatory process. The process is designed to be used by the range of mental health professionals working within school or community contexts. Because of the unique position of school psychologists as mental health specialists with expertise in school-based psychological practice, we pay particular attention to the skills they bring as facilitators of the PCSIM process. What is most critical is that the program planner brings together partners with the necessary expertise and knowledge.

PHASE 1: EXISTING THEORY, RESEARCH, AND PRACTICE (EXPLORING PERSONAL THEORY)

The key considerations for Phase 1 are outlined in Exhibit 4.1. The primary goal of Phase 1 is to identify the theories, research, and professional

EXHIBIT 4.1
Key Considerations for Phase 1: Existing Theory, Research, and Practice (Personal Theory)

Focus (key questions)—Why?

- How do personal or professional views, knowledge, and experience influence definitions of mental health (mental problems/illness) and strategies for promoting mental health (reducing risk, treating mental illness)?
- What is the purpose for our collaboration?
- What are the initial concerns or reasons for program development?

Participants—Who?

- Program planner or planners (researcher, interventionist, consultant)
- Professionals with expertise in relevant theories and research
- Representatives of potential partners (stakeholders)

Tasks or Activities—What?

- Gather data about stakeholder concerns and worldviews related to children's mental health
- Gain self-understanding of personal theory related to children's mental health
- Establish relationships with potential partners and representatives of relevant stakeholder groups
- Gain entry into the target contexts, organizations, communities
- Review and share with stakeholders or partners professional literature on mental health to facilitate theory–research–practice links

Strategies or Methods—How?

- Conduct meetings with stakeholder groups
- Conduct informal contacts with potential partners and key informants (who are knowledgeable about culture, context, or mental health issues)
- Conduct participant observation in relevant contexts (e.g., schools, classrooms, community settings)
- Engage in reflection regarding one's own personal theory
- Conduct individual or group interviews and surveys with stakeholders to determine concerns, interests, and personal and professional perspectives regarding children's mental health

Requisite Skills (potential focus for staff recruitment and training)

- Reflective practice or personal reflection
- Communication (sharing information, expressing self, listening, eliciting views, negotiation of perspectives)
- Ethnographic techniques (data collection, analysis, interpretation)
- Reviewing and summarizing professional literature on mental health for dissemination to various stakeholder groups
- Expertise in mental health promotion, including program development, implementation, and evaluation of mental health programs ranging from prevention to treatment

Challenges

- Engage in ongoing process of self-reflection (monitoring personal perspective, bias, etc.) or reflective practice (linking research and theory with practice)
- Gain access to insights of others by promoting reflection, asking right questions, and establishing trust
- Deal with discrepant perspectives or personal theories; integrate divergent views and build consensus among partners

(continued)

EXHIBIT 4.1   *(Continued)*

Opportunities

- Establish trust with partners or stakeholders early in the process of program development
- Initiate partnerships by engaging stakeholders in early stages of program development
- Foster involvement, commitment, ownership, and empowerment among stakeholders
- Enhance awareness of one's own personal theories
- Acquire knowledge of personal theories of other partners or stakeholders
- Educate stakeholders about the potential links of theory and research to meeting the mental health needs of the target population

and personal experiences that influence program planners and stakeholders. In addition, this phase provides the context for initial discussion of the purpose of the proposed collaboration, whether to plan a comprehensive program or specific interventions. From this initial phase, the program planner engages representatives from the key stakeholder groups and potential partners. It behooves program planners to conduct formal and informal interactions with stakeholders from the beginning in a manner that fosters trust and provides a context for discussing issues and concerns in the language[2] of the stakeholders. Strategies for identifying and engaging partners in a participatory process are discussed in the context of Phase 3, Forming Partnerships. In this section, we focus on the elicitation of personal theories.

Personal theory refers to the theoretical or philosophical perspective that guides the work and actions of individuals. Personal theory is continuously evolving and represents the accumulated integration of education, professional experience, and personal and cultural experiences into a coherent framework for making sense of the world. This definition is consistent with that suggested by Brammer, Shostrom, and Abrego (1989) to describe personal theory building by professional therapists and counselors.

The identification of the theoretical–empirical basis that guides the work of the program planner is an extension of the formal process that precedes science-based research and practice. That is, the professional identifies the relevant theoretical and empirical foundations through systematic review of the relevant literature base and through consideration of the theoretical–empirical foundations that usually guide his or her work. For example, the foundations of the conceptual model that guided the Sri Lanka Mental Health (SLMH) Project (see Figure 3.3, chap. 3, this volume)

---

[2] The term *language* as used here refers to the meaning and vocabulary in a broad sense. Even in interactions between professionals, eliciting the meaning of terminology is essential to ensuring accurate understanding and clarity.

included ecological–developmental theory (Bronfenbrenner, 1989), the interaction of self- and interpersonal development (Guisinger & Blatt, 1994; Harter, 1999), existing models of individual and community mental health (e.g., Elias & Branden, 1988), and our previous work in mental health promotion (e.g., Nastasi & DeZolt, 1994).

The personal theories of professionals and nonprofessionals are likely to come from different sources. Although professional planners and stakeholders are expected to draw from existing theory and research and their professional experiences, it also is necessary that they examine their own personal viewpoints and experiences that influence their approach to practice. In addition, they have the responsibility to facilitate examination of the worldviews and experiences that influence how the various nonprofessional stakeholders perceive mental health needs and resources.

Specific strategies for identifying and articulating personal theories of planners and stakeholders are summarized in Exhibit 4.2. Before guiding partners and other stakeholders in the process of articulation, we suggest that mental health professionals (individually or collectively) use the following process to explicate their own understanding and practice related to mental health of children and adolescents.

1. Review the theoretical, empirical, and clinical–applied literature on children and adolescent mental health and mental health promotion, with reference to the continuum of prevention to treatment. Use this as a basis for articulating your own perspective on what constitutes mental health, what factors influence mental health, and effective strategies for promoting mental health or treating mental health problems or illness.

2. Examine your own practice with regard to mental health assessment and intervention (along the continuum of prevention to treatment) with school-age populations, asking questions such as the following:
   a. What *constructs* are included in the assessment and intervention tools that you use?
   b. To what extent do you *focus* on the emotional, cognitive, and behavioral functioning of the child or adolescent?
   c. To what extent do you address *cultural* and *contextual factors* related to family, school, peer group, and community?
   d. What *methods* (observations, interviews, self-reports, standardized tests) and *sources* (child, parent, teacher) do you use to gather data about child or adolescent functioning?
   e. What *prevention, risk reduction, intervention,* and *treatment approaches* do you use to address the mental health needs of children and adolescents? What have you found to be

EXHIBIT 4.2
Strategies for Eliciting and Articulating Personal Theories

Personal Reflections for Program Planners
- Engage in a reflective process prior to meeting with stakeholders to identify the theoretical and empirical bases that guide your approach to assessment and intervention.
- Describe how you typically approach assessment and intervention within a practical setting.
- Describe how you typically approach a research problem.
- Define key concepts such as *mental health, mental illness, prevention,* and *treatment.*
- Identify what you consider to be appropriate goals for school-based mental health and appropriate roles for various stakeholders.
- Articulate what you know about the target population—where they live, their language, values, customs, and so on.
- Identify what you value—what is most important to you—as a person and professional.

Identifying Stakeholders' Theories
- Engage in participant observation in the target context; for example, visit the school and classrooms, attend school and community events, and interact informally with stakeholders.
- Conduct focus groups (or meetings) with representatives of the different stakeholder groups to identify their primary concerns, how they view their role and your role, what they view as possible solutions. Conduct these meetings in a context that is familiar to stakeholders. Look for patterns of similarity and difference across individuals and groups. Conduct meetings with separate stakeholder groups as well as with representatives across groups.
- Conduct individual interviews with representatives of stakeholder groups to elicit personal perspectives, values, concerns, and beliefs.
- Conduct brief surveys with a larger cross-section of stakeholders. Include questions that parallel the focus groups and individual interviews.
- Facilitate discussion among stakeholders to identify similarities and differences in perspective and facilitate negotiation of perspectives, to determine potential points of consensus as well as issues that are likely to remain contentious.

most effective, and why? What factors account for variations in effectiveness; for example, type or severity of problem, developmental level of child or adolescent, involvement of significant others in assessment and intervention, length of the intervention, use of individual versus group approaches, direct versus indirect service delivery?

3. Describe the theoretical perspective (e.g., what single theory or integration of several theories) that guides how you (a) conceptualize mental health and (b) approach mental health intervention with children and adolescents.

The identification of personal theories is likely to take time and continues throughout the PCSIM process through reflection; dialogue; ongoing data collection, analysis, and interpretation; and attempts to negotiate multiple perspectives and reach consensus on key issues related to program development. Activities of Phase 2 (Learning the Culture) are particularly helpful for eliciting stakeholders' personal theories. For example, questions posed to stakeholders for the purposes of exploring cultural norms, beliefs, values, language, and practices also elicit personal theories. Although we present Phases 1 and 2 separately, in practice the methods and activities of these two phases are likely to overlap.

PHASE 2: LEARNING THE CULTURE

The focus of Phase 2 activities is the understanding of cultural similarities and differences among stakeholder groups regarding conceptions of mental health and mental health promotion (see Exhibit 4.3). *Culture* refers to the shared (or common) values, beliefs, ideas, norms, and language of the members of a particular culture (e.g., group, community, organization, society) as well as the individual interpretations of cultural experiences. The purpose of *ethnography* is to understand culture from the perspective of members of a particular group, community, or society. Ethnographers attempt to gain an *emic* perspective, that is, the point of view of the insiders or those being studied (in contrast to the *etic* or outside perspective of the researcher).

We propose that ethnographic methods (see Table 2.2, chap. 2, this volume) provide the mechanism for understanding the personal theories of stakeholders as well as for understanding the range of cultures they are likely to represent. We also have used these methods successfully to study cultures in other countries (e.g., Nastasi et al., 1998–1999; Nastasi, Varjas, Sarkar, & Jayasena, 1998). Using participant observation, focus groups, and individual interviews, one can come to understand the personal theories and cultural experiences of parents, teachers, students, administrators, other school staff, community agency staff, and community members. Specific strategies for identifying stakeholders' personal theories are outlined in Exhibit 4.2. Questions to guide data collection with stakeholders that cover both personal theories and culture include the following:

1. What are the conceptions (definitions) of mental health, mental health problems, and mental illness held by various stakeholders? What language (vocabulary) do they use to talk about mental health or mental illness or related constructs (e.g., dysfunction, adjustment difficulties, behavior problems)?
2. What mental health outcomes are valued by stakeholders?
3. What influences the mental health (well-being, school adjustment, etc.) of children and adolescents?

EXHIBIT 4.3
Key Considerations for Phase 2: Learning the Culture

Focus (key questions)—Why?

- What are the shared (and discrepant) language, values, beliefs, norms, and practices related to definitions of mental health (target concern)?
- What mental health outcomes (outcomes related to target concern) are socially valued?
- What social–cultural factors influence child and adolescent mental health (target concern)?

Participants—Who?

- Program planner or planners (researcher, interventionist, consultant)
- Professionals with expertise in study of culture or ethnographic techniques
- Representatives of all stakeholder groups

Tasks or Activities—What?

- Study the culture of target groups, ethnographic data collection, analysis, and interpretation
- Develop relationships with partners and representatives of stakeholder groups
- Gain entry into target contexts, organizations, communities
- Identify potential partners and cultural brokers (who can facilitate access and interpret culture)

Strategies or Methods—How?

- Engage in multimethod (individual or group interviews, focus groups, surveys, collect records or artifacts), multisource (representatives of key stakeholder groups) data collection to study culture of target groups and identify socially valued mental health outcomes and culture-specific social–cultural influences on mental health
- Engage in informal contacts with potential partners and key informants (who are knowledgeable about culture, context, or mental health issues)
- Conduct participant observation in relevant contexts (e.g., schools, community settings)

Requisite Skills (potential focus for recruitment and training)

- Ethnography—data collection, analysis, interpretation, dissemination
- Interpersonal skills for developing partnerships and negotiating relationships with stakeholders
- Organizational consultation, systems change, capacity-building skills
- Ecological perspective and approach to research and intervention

Challenges

- Gain acceptance of various stakeholders
- Build trust with stakeholders, partners, cultural brokers
- Go beyond etic (outsider) perspective of the researchers–planners to achieve understanding of emic (insider) perspective of stakeholders or consumers

Opportunities

- Foster involvement, commitment, and ownership among stakeholders
- Identify cultural brokers who can interpret the culture of and provide critical links to key stakeholders and contexts
- Assess feasibility of mental health programming
- Gain emic perspective of various partners or stakeholders regarding factors related to mental health promotion

4. To what extent can adults (e.g., parents, teachers) and peers influence the mental health of children and adolescents? Who has responsibility for ensuring the psychological well-being of children?
5. What are the common problems that children and adolescents exhibit in school? In the community? At home?
6. What kinds of experiences at school, at home, or in the community are likely to put children and adolescents at risk for mental health (school adjustment) problems?
7. How do the school, family, and community respond to mental health issues of students? What resources or programs are currently available in the school or community?
8. What can schools do to promote mental health of students? What kinds of programs or approaches are likely to work best for students in this school or community?

It may be beneficial for program planners to ask themselves these same questions as a way to gauge consistencies and discrepancies among partners.

Analyses of the ethnographic data are focused on identifying themes with regard to the mental health–illness continuum, vocabulary relevant to mental health, culturally valued mental health outcomes, perceived factors that influence mental health, perceived stakeholder responsibilities and roles, and possible intervention strategies across the continuum of prevention to treatment. In analyzing data, planners give particular attention to the range of responses and points of agreement and disagreement. These themes, along with the conceptual model of the program planner and alternative models from the literature, are presented to the representatives of the various stakeholder groups for feedback and discussion. The purpose of presentation and discussion is to promote understanding of the diversity of perspectives and work toward a shared framework and vocabulary for approaching mental health programming. Such discussion also can help program planners to identify similarities and discrepancies between their perspectives and those of stakeholders, and to enhance their own understanding of culture-specific conceptions.

The interview questions in Exhibit 4.4 were used in a school-based drug and sexual risk prevention program for middle school students[3] to assess

---

[3] A 4½-year intervention research project, "Building Preventive Group Norms in Urban Middle Schools," funded by the National Institute on Drug Abuse, National Institutes of Health (Grant No. DA12015; Jean Schensul, principal investigator, Institute for Community Research, Hartford, Connecticut; Bonnie K. Nastasi, co-principal investigator, Institute for Community Research; and David Schonfeld, co-principal investigator, Yale University). The project involves the development, implementation, and evaluation of classroom-based interventions that focus on developing peer norms to support healthy decisions regarding drug use and adolescent sexual relationships. The program targets sixth- and seventh-grade students.

EXHIBIT 4.4
In-Depth Interview Questions for Teachers of Middle School Students

1. Tell me about your experience with teaching a social–emotional development curriculum?
   (If the teacher has experience with existing curriculum): What do you think about the existing curriculum?
   (If the teacher has not had experience with existing curriculum): Have you heard about the social–emotional development curriculum? Why haven't you used it?
2. Tell me about your experience using cooperative learning? What do you think about it?
   If you haven't used it, have you done small group work with students? What do you think are appropriate goals for cooperative learning?
3. What do you think of combining social–emotional development and cooperative learning?
4. What are key social and emotional issues for your students? How are these manifested in the classroom?
5. What kinds of discipline problems do you face with students? How do you handle these?
6. What do you think about prevention programs for social, emotional, or health risks (i.e., drugs, sexual risk)?
7. Describe your approach to teaching. (Probe for teaching philosophy, experiences, training)
8. What training have you received regarding social–emotional development of students? What training have you received in cooperative learning?
9. What is an appropriate role for teachers regarding students' social and emotional development? Teaching students about drugs? Teaching about reproductive health and sexual risks?
10. In addition to teaching a social–emotional curriculum, how do you address social development or social issues in the classroom? Where else in the curriculum do you include objectives related to social and emotional development, drugs, reproductive health, or sexual risks (e.g., pregnancy, sexually transmitted diseases, HIV)? What would you like to change about your current approach? What can the school do differently to address students' personal and interpersonal problems and social issues?

Note. These interview questions were designed for use in a 4½-year intervention-research project, "Building Preventive Group Norms in Urban Middle Schools," funded by the National Institute on Drug Abuse, National Institutes of Health (Grant No. DA12015; Jean Schensul, principal investigator, Institute for Community Research, Hartford, Connecticut; Bonnie K. Nastasi, co-principal investigator, Institute for Community Research; and David Schonfeld, Yale University). The project involves the development, implementation, and evaluation of classroom-based interventions (with sixth and seventh graders) that focus on developing peer norms to support healthy decisions regarding drug use and adolescent sexual relationships.

participating teachers' philosophy, preparation, knowledge, attitudes, beliefs, and practices related to their role in addressing students' social and emotional difficulties, health risks such as drug and sexual risks, and social issues such as violence. These interviews were semistructured and included general questions, with additional questions to probe for specific information. This format permitted standardization with flexibility for individual variations. Interview responses provided data about teachers' personal theories, acceptability of program components, and staff development needs. These questions guided data collection before program implementation to assess initial perspectives and needs, during implementation to monitor program acceptability and staff development needs, and after implementation to evaluate changes in teacher perspectives.

Phase 1 and 2 activities also provide the foundation for identifying program goals or specific stakeholder concerns during Phase 4. As noted earlier, Phases 1 through 3 are likely to coincide with entry into the system and negotiation of the purpose of coming together. Critical to these early phases as well as throughout the PCSIM process are partnerships with those who have vested interests and necessary resources related to mental health programming. In the next section, we describe the procedures for achieving effective partnerships.

PHASE 3: FORMING PARTNERSHIPS

The participatory process of PCSIM necessitates the involvement of key stakeholders as partners in the development of comprehensive school-based mental health programs. As indicated in Exhibit 4.5, the focus of Phase 3 is to identify and engage stakeholders and establish a process for working together effectively. We propose the use of a *participatory consultation model* (described in chap. 2, this volume, and Nastasi, Varjas, Bernstein, & Jayasena, 2000) to involve stakeholders in a team process of co-constructing interventions. *Essential to the success of participatory problem solving and decision making are the communication and negotiation skills of all partners*. Training in these skills is critical to effective team functioning.

In this section, we describe a model of group process that addresses both participant and facilitator skills. We have used this model successfully in conducting research, providing training, and facilitating group process across a range of populations (including children, adolescents, community members, teachers, and other professionals). First, however, we address the issue of identifying and securing partners.

Partners

Potential participants in the development of comprehensive school-based mental health programs include professionals who have relevant expertise or provide existing mental health services in the school or local community agency as well as professionals or paraprofessionals who can assist in program delivery, provide necessary resources, or represent consumers of services. Program planners are encouraged to assemble an interdisciplinary team with expertise in mental health theory, research, practice, and training. Such professionals can be found within the school system, local community

EXHIBIT 4.5
Key Considerations for Phase 3: Forming Partnerships

Focus (key questions)—Why?
- Who are the key stakeholder groups?
- Who are the cultural brokers?
- How do we engage stakeholders?
- How do we work together effectively?

Participants—Who?
- Program planner or planners (researcher, interventionist, consultant)
- Professionals with expertise in systems change, organizational consultation, team or group process
- Representatives of key stakeholder groups
- Potential cultural brokers (who can facilitate access and interpret culture)
- Primary partners

Tasks or Activities—What?
- Bring partners together
- Establish participatory structure and process

Strategies or Methods—How?
- Collaborative–participatory consultation
- Group facilitation or team building

Requisite Skills (potential focus for recruitment and training)
- Collaboration, team building, group problem solving
- Group facilitation skills
- Group process evaluation
- Leadership

Challenges
- Overcome existing hierarchical structure or orientation of system to establish equitable partnership roles
- Address role expectations for partners
- Address individuals' need for control and foster sharing of responsibilities
- Overcome preference for expert approach to program development
- Identify relevant strengths of partners and engage them accordingly (empowerment)

Opportunities
- Promote stakeholder involvement, ownership, and empowerment
- Establish a sustainable participatory process

agencies, colleges and universities, and research institutes. Although national or regional experts can be enlisted, it is advisable to draw on local experts who can make sustained contributions and support capacity building. Potential mental health specialists include psychologists, psychiatrists, social workers, and counselors. Prospective research partners include psychologists, anthropologists, sociologists, and educational, medical, and public health researchers. Also important are other school-based professionals whose involvement is critical to planning, implementing, or sustaining programs.

These include, for example, district- and building-level administrators, classroom teachers, special education personnel, curriculum developers, health educators, drug education specialists, and police, truancy, and security officers. To facilitate interagency partnerships, program planners need to invite professionals working in local government or private social service agencies such as hospitals, mental health centers, child protection agencies, police departments, parole offices, and juvenile court. Assembling an interdisciplinary and interagency team is a daunting task but is essential to the development and maintenance of comprehensive service delivery.

Nonprofessional partners include school and community stakeholders whose involvement is critical to program success. These include those who, with training and supervision, can assist in components of program delivery as paraprofessionals (e.g., helping with intervention, outreach, parent involvement); those who can support program efforts (e.g., by providing funds, contributing equipment and materials, or assisting in transportation of students, building maintenance, or clerical tasks); and those who constitute the consumers or recipients of services (e.g., students and parents).

In theory, partners include all those individuals who play critical roles within the ecology of the child, including the school, home, and community (e.g., parents, teachers, community members). In practice, partners who are engaged in the PCSIM process are representatives of these various stakeholder groups. Over the course of programming efforts, the cast of players changes. Some individuals invest considerable time and effort throughout the process and constitute a core team. Others assist in limited ways or for limited periods of time depending on their interest and the needs of the program.

Critical to system entry and cultural interpretation is a partner we refer to as the *cultural broker* (Nastasi, Varjas, Bernstein, & Jayasena, 2000). As we described in chapter 3, the cultural broker serves as both the expert on the culture of the target population (e.g., students, community members) and the liaison to the target context or community (e.g., school system, social service community, local neighborhood). Given the scope of comprehensive mental health programming and the range of stakeholder groups, it is likely that program planners will establish relationships with several cultural brokers.

Participatory Problem Solving and Decision Making

Essential to the successful involvement of stakeholders as partners in program development is a participatory approach to problem solving and decision making. This process involves engaging partners in (a) identifying goals (or problems); (b) brainstorming strategies (solutions); (c) evaluating the potential effectiveness of suggested strategies (i.e., consequences,

EXHIBIT 4.6
Participatory Problem Solving and Decision Making:
Steps and Key Questions

Step 1: Goal or problem description
What is the goal (or problem)?

Step 2: Brainstorm strategies or solutions
What are possible courses of action?

Step 3: Consider and evaluate each strategy
What are potential consequences?
What factors (people, conditions, resources) would facilitate carrying out the strategy?
What factors pose barriers to carrying out the strategy?
Would the strategy (solution) work? Why or why not?

Step 4: Choose a strategy or solution
Given your answers to questions in Step 3, which strategy or combination of strategies is most likely to be feasible and effective?

Step 5: Action plan
What needs to be done? What is the plan of action?
How will the plan be carried out? What are the steps or actions?
Who will be involved? And what roles and responsibilities will they have?
Where will it happen?
When will the plan be implemented? How long will it take?

Step 6: Evaluation plan
How will we determine whether the plan is acceptable to those who will either carry it out or be affected by it?
How will we monitor implementation of the plan?
How will we determine if the plan of action is effective?
What specific evaluation activities need to occur?
Who will be involved in conducting the activities?
What is the timeline for conducting evaluation activities?
How will we use evaluation data to foster success of the action plan?

facilitators, barriers); (d) selecting a general strategy; (e) developing a plan of action (identifying players, responsibilities, location, and timeline); and (f) developing a plan for monitoring and evaluation (see Exhibit 4.6). The underlying assumptions are that divergent viewpoints are expected and valued, and that the goal is to achieve consensus about a plan of action. Critical to the success of this participatory process are skills such as relationship building, communication (expressing ideas, active listening, questioning, clarification), brainstorming, eliciting divergent ideas, consideration and discussion of alternative viewpoints, reaching a mutually agreeable outcome (i.e., consensus), and self-evaluation (of the participatory process). Exhibit 4.7 provides an outline of critical group process skills.

The responsibility of the program planners is to establish the structure and process for participatory problem solving and decision making. This involves bringing partners together to work in teams of six to eight members, providing training, arranging for group facilitators, setting the schedule

EXHIBIT 4.7
Critical Skills for Participatory Problem Solving and Decision Making

Building Relationships

- Getting to know each other
- Identifying common interests
- Communicating ideas
- Communicating feelings
- Responding to others' needs
- Roles in groups
- Rules for working together—setting rules, monitoring, revising
- Group responsibility—individual and group accountability

Communication

- Presenting ideas
- Listening to others
- Asking questions
- Answering questions
- Checking for meaning
- Rephrasing
- Summarizing
- Nonverbal cues

Collaborative Problem Solving

- Each person identifies feelings
- Each person states the problem and identifies a goal
- Brainstorm solutions together
- Consider consequences of each solution
- Choose a solution everyone agrees on

Consensus Building

- Seeking ideas from others
- Brainstorming
- Recording ideas
- Perspective taking—seeing another's point of view
- Discussing and considering each person's ideas
- Learning ways to reach agreement

Resolving Dilemmas

- Respecting different points of view
- Seeking different points of view
- Trying to understand another's viewpoint
- Accepting another person's point of view
- Finding middle ground
- Combining different ideas so all views are reflected

Self-Evaluation

- Identifying the outcome of the group process
- Determining if the group was successful
- Identifying the strategies used by group members that helped or hindered the group process
- Generating ideas to improve group process

of team meetings, and developing a system of group self-evaluation. The facilitation of the group process involves setting ground rules, posing questions, eliciting responses, monitoring participation to ensure equitable contributions by group members, keeping the discussion on topic, recording and summarizing key points, helping group members combine similar ideas and synthesize discrepant ideas, checking for understanding and agreement, intervening when disagreements become personal, securing commitment to the plan of action, and guiding a discussion about the quality and success of the group process. (For additional information on facilitating professional collaboration and team process in school settings, see Friend & Cook, 1996; Rosenfield & Gravois, 1996.)

The participatory process is highly dependent on the extent to which stakeholders can engage in the interpersonal process of group decision making. It behooves program planners to approach the team process in a systematic manner, to invest time in training and monitoring the team process, and to solicit assistance from expert facilitators or arrange for training of in-house facilitators. The success and sustainability of the team process is a key element of institutionalization and capacity building. As with all aspects of staff development, we recommend conducting staff training on group process using a consultation approach in which initial training sessions are followed by a series of additional training (booster) sessions and on-site support to monitor implementation and provide individualized assistance.

PHASE 4: GOAL OR PROBLEM IDENTIFICATION

Phase 4 is devoted to more clearly articulating the purpose for the application of PCSIM. In practice, the identification of goals or concerns that will guide program development efforts began in Phase 1. Phase 4 is best considered as an outgrowth of the activities of Phases 1 through 3, as well as the impetus for Phases 5 and 6, which are devoted to achieving a more in-depth understanding of the target phenomenon (i.e., goal or problem) and the influential or mediating factors that can serve as additional targets for intervention. The primary activities of Phase 4 (see Exhibit 4.8) are preparing the information gathered in Phases 1 and 2 for review by stakeholders and conducting a participatory decision-making process to review data, clarify the goal(s) for program development, and identify questions to guide the formative research of Phase 5. It is important to avoid artificial segmentation of the phases of PCSIM. In practice, phase activities overlap, and the process is seamless and iterative. What is essential is that program planners (and ultimately stakeholders) remain cognizant of and monitor the progression through the 12 critical components of PCSIM (as depicted in Figures 3.1 and 3.2, chap. 3, this volume).

EXHIBIT 4.8
Key Considerations for Phase 4: Goal or Problem Identification

Focus (key questions)—Why?
- What are the target concerns (problems) to be addressed?
- What are the program goals (desired outcomes)?

Participants—Who?
- Program planner or planners (researcher, interventionist, consultant)
- Professionals with expertise in organizational consultation, systems change, group process
- Cultural brokers (who can facilitate access and interpret culture)
- Representatives of stakeholder groups

Tasks or Activities—What?
- Examine data from Phases 1 and 2, in partnership with stakeholders
- Reach consensus among partners or stakeholders on target concern or goal
- Identify questions for formative research phase

Strategies or Methods—How?
- Participatory problem solving or consensus building
- Facilitation of participatory process

Requisite Skills (potential focus for recruitment and training)
- Participatory problem-solving skills—communication, negotiation, consensus building
- Group facilitation skills (e.g., engaging participants in idea generation, ensuring equitable participation, guiding group toward consensus)
- Ability to articulate problem or goals in terms that are acceptable, socially valid, achievable, and reflect integration of divergent perspectives

Challenges
- Deal with discrepant perspectives on problem or goal; integrate divergent views and build consensus among partners
- Overcome existing hierarchical structure or orientation of system to establish equitable participation across various stakeholders
- Overcome preference for expert approach to program development
- Address potential barriers posed by existing interpersonal relationships (e.g., extant conflicts, cliques, political camps)
- Foster equity across stakeholder groups

Opportunities
- Promote stakeholder involvement, ownership, and empowerment
- Establish a sustainable participatory problem-solving and consensus-building process
- Foster explication of concerns and goals from multiple perspectives
- Reach agreement on common goal(s) or shared mission
- Foster partnership across stakeholder groups

PHASE 5: FORMATIVE RESEARCH

The primary purpose of Phase 5 is to conduct systematic research on the target phenomena related to the goal(s) of program development. In Exhibit 4.9, we list the key questions for framing the research process. The

EXHIBIT 4.9
Key Considerations for Phase 5: Formative Research

Focus (key questions)—Why?

- What psychological, social–cultural, and environmental factors influence mental health (or the specific constructs of interest); that is, what are the factors that mediate mental health for the target population?
- How are key constructs (mental health and mediating factors) defined within the target culture?
- What are the nature and prevalence of mental health problems (target concerns) in target population or culture?
- What personal, social–cultural, and environmental (physical, structural, economic) resources are available within the target context(s)?
- What are the facilitators and barriers to change (prevention or intervention) efforts?

Participants—Who?

- Program planner or planners (researcher, interventionist, consultant)
- Professional(s) with expertise in qualitative and quantitative research methods
- Professional(s) with expertise in mental health research and practice
- Cultural brokers (who can facilitate access and interpret culture)
- Representatives of stakeholder groups

Tasks or Activities—What?

- Educate stakeholders about importance, process, and methods of formative research (for data-based decision making)
- Select or develop research instruments
- Data collection and analysis
- Data interpretation and member checking

Strategies or Methods—How?

- Engage in multimethod (see list that follows), multisource (representatives of various stakeholder groups) data collection to define culture-specific individual and cultural constructs related to mental health; identify culture-specific mental health needs and resources; and identify potential facilitators and barriers to mental health programming. Specific techniques include (see Table 2.2, chap. 2, this volume, for definitions):
  - Naturalistic or participant observation
  - Individual and group interviews
  - Focus groups
  - Ethnographic surveys
  - Self- and informant reports
  - Records, archives, artifacts
  - Logs, journals, narratives
  - Social network and spatial mapping
  - Elicitation (e.g., freelists, pilesorts)

Requisite Skills (potential focus for recruitment and training)

- Relevant research skills (i.e., expertise in multimethod, multisource data collection, analysis, interpretation; skill in relevant research techniques)
- Participatory problem-solving skills—communication, negotiation, consensus building
- Group facilitation skills (e.g., engaging participants in idea generation, ensuring equitable participation, guiding group toward consensus)

(continued)

EXHIBIT 4.9 *(Continued)*

Challenges

- Secure individuals with relevant research expertise
- Promote acceptability of research process among stakeholders
- Achieve commitment of necessary time and effort from stakeholders

Opportunities

- Ensure ecological validity and cultural specificity of mental health programs
- Achieve in-depth understanding of phenomena or problems of interest
- Engage in data-based approach to decision making and program planning
- Develop research skills and appreciation for research application among stakeholders
- Build research capacity within the target contexts (e.g., agency, community)

outcome of this phase is the articulation of a culture-specific conceptual model that depicts the target construct (e.g., general mental health or specific mental health issue such as depression or attention deficit hyperactivity disorder) and the relevant mediating factors (e.g., stressors, resources, cultural norms). In addition, formative research is directed toward understanding the nature and scope of the phenomenon of interest (e.g., How is depression manifested in this adolescent population? What is the incidence of depression in this community?). Moreover, data collection is directed toward the identification of facilitators (e.g., available resources, cultural norms, socialization practices) and barriers (e.g., lack of funds, poorly integrated services, denial of depression as an adolescent problem) that are likely to influence programming efforts (e.g., to reduce the risk of adolescent depression or to establish effective screening procedures). In our own work, for example, the conceptual model identified in Phase 1 (see Figure 3.3, chap. 3, this volume) was the foundation for formative research in one community of Sri Lanka that culminated in the development of a culture-specific mental health promotion program and culture-specific assessment tools for program evaluation (Nastasi, Varjas, Bernstein, & Jayasena, 2000; Nastasi, Varjas, Sarkar, & Jayasena, 1998).

The action research process and ethnographic methods that are foundational to PCSIM provide the methodology for conducting Phase 5 activities. Phase 5 is an outgrowth of earlier phases. The general questions about key constructs and mediating factors that guide data collection in Phases 1 and 2 activities are applicable to Phase 5. Moreover, the data collection techniques are similar to those used in Phases 1 and 2. Despite these similarities, Phase 5 activities are distinct in several ways. First, the formative research of Phase 5 is more focused as a result of Phase 1 through 4 activities. Second, data collection involves a more in-depth exploration of key constructs. That is, Phase 5 data collection provides the opportunity to confirm, disconfirm, and elaborate on initial (Phase 1–2) findings or assumptions.

Third, Phase 5 formative research encompasses a larger and more representative sample of the stakeholder populations. Fourth, Phase 5 research involves the use of a broader set of methods and more intensive research process. Thus, the formative research process of Phase 5, in contrast to initial data-gathering activities of Phases 1 and 2, is more time-intensive and has greater depth and scope. Moreover, Phase 5 has a different purpose, that is, to create a culture-specific (local) conceptual framework to guide intervention and capacity-building activities of subsequent phases. Whereas Phases 1 and 2 might be considered exploratory in nature, Phase 5 constitutes in-depth investigation guided by the initial framework constructed from the earlier exploration.

Inherent in PCSIM are an anthropological–ethnographic perspective and the use of mixed methods (i.e., qualitative and quantitative) for data collection and analysis. In chapter 2, we described an ethnographic perspective and research and evaluation methods applicable to conducting school-based interventions. With the exception of a few (e.g., pilesorts, freelists), the ethnographic techniques used in this phase are consistent with data collection strategies used by school psychologists in conducting psychological evaluations and consultation. For example, school psychologists typically make use of observations, interviews, records review, and student, teacher, and parent reports. These techniques are often viewed as informal and lacking standardization. The ethnographic approach is designed to formalize and systematize the collection, analysis, and integration of data obtained through such methods. In addition, the participatory approach is aimed toward educating and involving stakeholders in the research and evaluation activities, thus helping to build institutional capacity. Furthermore, the data are used in a systematic way to design interventions tailored to the local context and population, thus promoting sustainability and institutionalization.

Although the formative research phase is best completed prior to program development, there are instances in which in-depth data collection is not feasible. In a school-based drug abuse prevention project currently under way (see Footnote 3), it was not possible (because of funding restraints and organizational restrictions) to conduct a formative research phase prior to program development. Planners relied on information from staff members who were responsible for monitoring and supporting the existing drug prevention program. In the context of implementation, data collected for program monitoring and evaluation purposes indicated that some aspects of the program lacked cultural specificity. Using these data, program planners proposed and subsequently implemented formative research activities conducted simultaneously with program implementation. For example, students were interviewed about their experiences related to drug risks using procedures that were separate from classroom-based curriculum activities. Critical to securing permission for these research activities were the relationships developed with the system administrators and staff and the data-based justification (i.e., evidence from evaluation data collected within the system).

Phase 5 activities involve the selection and design of data collection tools and the coordination of data collection, analysis, and interpretation in preparation for the development of local theory and action plans. Just as Phases 1 and 2 lead to the identification of goals or problems in Phase 4, Phase 5 leads to the development of a local theory in Phase 6 and the design of programs in Phase 7.

Illustration

We exemplify Phase 5 activities using a hypothetical urban school district with initial concerns related to school and community violence, depression and anxiety among students, availability of drugs in the community and on school campuses, and incidence of sexually transmitted diseases among high school students. A research and evaluation team has assumed responsibility for planning and implementing data collection throughout the PCSIM process. The team begins by exploring the availability of reliable archival school and district data on incidences of community and school violence, drug possession, and discipline referrals related to bullying. In addition, the school health and mental health staff are asked to provide summary information from their files on types of mental health concerns (e.g., depression, anxiety, aggression) and health-related issues such as drug abuse, pregnancy, and sexually transmitted diseases.

To assess the perceptions of school staff, students, and parents regarding the need for and potential scope of school-based mental health services, program planners initially approach the school principal to gather information about perceived mental health needs within the building, existing building-level or district-level services (e.g., availability of psychologists, social workers, counselors), access to services in the community, and emerging or unmet needs of students (e.g., incidents of sexual harassment and bullying of students, difficulty in addressing suicidal ideation or attempts, increase in number of students reporting drug use on a systemwide anonymous survey). The principal is asked to identify individuals within the building who have information about these concerns, for example, school nurse, seventh-grade teacher, school disciplinarian, and clinician in the school-based health clinic. As these informants are interviewed, they provide additional or conflicting information and suggest additional informants (e.g., other teachers, drug educator from a community organization, and reproductive health educator from a local hospital). This process is repeated, in individual or group format, with representatives of parents and students. For example, a member of the planning team attends parent meetings at several schools to assess parental concerns and to identify individuals for follow-up interviews.

The outcomes of the series of key-informant interviews are (a) identification of key informants representing different stakeholder groups who can participate in later phases, (b) data about the range and scope of mental health concerns across the stakeholder groups, and (c) direction for more focused and in-depth data collection. During subsequent phases of PCSIM, key-informant interviews are used to help monitor reactions to the program, identify concerns as they arise, assess unintended effects, and maintain relationships with key stakeholders.

Using Ethnographic Methods for Conducting Formative Research

In this section, we provide examples of the application of ethnographic methods in the formative (research) phases of school-based intervention programs. In particular, we illustrate the use of focus groups and in-depth interviews, spatial mapping, and elicitation techniques (defined in Table 2.2, chap. 2, this volume).

Focus Groups and In-Depth Interviews

In one project, we conducted 51 focus groups (i.e., semi-structured, in-depth group interviews), 33 with students and 18 with teachers, to gather formative data on the mental health needs and resources of adolescents. (Individual in-depth interviews were conducted with school administrators, teachers, and counselors in settings in which group interviews were not feasible.) Working with a child psychiatrist and teacher educator in Sri Lanka, we developed a set of general questions (Exhibit 4.10, reprinted from Nastasi, Varjas, Sarkar, & Jayasena, 1998) to facilitate exploration of culture-specific definitions of constructs relevant to the program's theoretical model (see Figure 3.3, chap. 3, this volume). We used the general questions to guide interviews with students and teachers until we achieved a point of data saturation (i.e., subsequent interviews with different groups failed to provide additional information). Using responses to the general questions, we identified a set of common problems and concerns (see Exhibit 4.10) that guided the next stage of interviewing. The second stage continued until we again achieved data saturation.

We coded the interview data using a combined deductive–inductive process (Nastasi, 1999). Our proposed theoretical model guided initial coding. When data did not fit predetermined categories, we generated new categories. This process continued until a culture-specific coding scheme was achieved (i.e., the scheme encompassed the cultural experiences and interpretations of the target group). Interrater agreement was established,

EXHIBIT 4.10
Questions That Guided Focus Group Interviews
With Students and Teachers

Student Interview Questions

General Questions

- Describe a good (not good) student.
- Describe a good (not good) friend.
- Describe a good (not good) citizen.
- Describe a good (not good) parent.
- Describe a good (not good) teacher.
- What makes children happy?
- What makes children sad or unhappy?
- What makes children angry?
- What makes children scared or frightened?
- What makes children confused?

Feelings (Emotions: happy, sad, angry, frightened, confused)

- What makes children or youths feel [emotion]?
- How can you tell if someone is feeling [emotion]?
- How do children or youths express [emotion]?
- What can someone do when feeling [emotion]?
- What can you do for a friend who is feeling [emotion]?

Common Problems (as indicated by respondents early in the interview process)

- Academic pressure or failure
- Test anxiety
- All study or no play
- Family is poor
- Alcoholic parent
- Mother in Middle East
- Break-up of love affair

Questions about common problems

- Do youths in Sri Lanka experience [problem]?
- How do youths feel in response to or about [problem]?
- What effect does [problem] have on youths?
- What do youths do about [problem]?
- Whom can youths talk to about [problem]?

Teacher Interview Questions

- Describe a good student. Describe a poor student.
- What skills or qualities do students need to do well in school? How important are social skills? Self-assurance?
- How do students express emotions?
- In what ways do students differ in academic ability? Social ability?
- Describe a good citizen. Describe a poor citizen.
- Who is responsible for preparing youths to be good citizens?
- Describe a good parent. Describe a poor parent.
- Describe a good teacher. Describe a poor teacher.
- How is discipline handled in the classroom or school? Who has the responsibility for discipline in the school?
- What types of rewards are used?

(continued)

EXHIBIT 4.10 *(Continued)*

- What problems do Sri Lankan youths experience in school? At home?
- Describe a student who is having problems.
- How can you tell a student in your classroom has a problem? What would or could you do about it?

Note. From "Participatory Model of Mental Health Programming: Lessons Learned From Work in a Developing Country," by B. K. Nastasi, K. Varjas, S. Sarkar, and A. Jayasena. 1998, *School Psychology Review,* *27,* p. 274. Copyright 1998 by the National Association of School Psychologists. Reprinted with permission.

and data were recoded with the culture-specific scheme. Results were interpreted in collaboration with Sri Lanka colleagues and stakeholders. Findings were used to (a) guide decision making about programming efforts in the district's schools, (b) develop a culture-specific assessment tool, and (c) develop a culture-specific mental health promotion curriculum (see Nastasi, Varjas, Sarkar, & Jayasena, 1998, for a detailed description of methods and findings).

What was particularly important about the approach was the opportunity to explore theoretical constructs based on work conducted in the United States (e.g., stressors, socially valued competencies, socialization practices) in the language of the participants and to develop tools that had cultural meaning in Sri Lanka. The stakeholders (professionals and community members) played key roles as partners in this process. These experiences underscored the value of considering culture-specific (local) meaning and the use of ethnographic methods for achieving this understanding. Moreover, these experiences subsequently influenced our approach to understanding health and mental health constructs in the United States.

Spatial Mapping

An example of the use of spatial mapping as a formative research tool comes from a study of high school violence by Astor, Meyer, and Behre (1999). The researchers used maps of school (all areas inside and outside of the building), semistructured interviews, and focus groups to investigate "the interaction of time and space within the social milieu of the high school" (Astor et al., 1999, p. 13). Students identified on the maps the locations where at least three violent events had occurred in the past year and places they considered to be unsafe or dangerous. For those locations where the violent events had occurred, the students were asked to indicate time of day when violence occurred, age and gender of participants in the violent incident or incidents, and the school's response to the incident. Maps were then used to facilitate focus group discussions to gather information about the nature of violent events and factors related to the perpetuation and prevention of violence (e.g., student–teacher relationships, gender, race, class, and specific interventions).

Using the data, Astor et al. (1999) generated "visual representation of specific hot spots for violence and dangerous time periods within each school" (p. 14). For example, the hot spots and times for older students were a parking lot after school; for younger students, lunchroom and hallways during transitions. Girls, compared with boys, reported more unsafe or dangerous areas, particularly in unsupervised locations. The coding of interview data revealed that most of the violent events were severe and potentially lethal. Student interview responses reflected a range of such events, including shootings or gun possession, stabbing, rape or sexual assault, and physical fights or assaults. Both student and staff informants suggested that the most violent locations were the "undefined spaces" that fell outside of the supervisory responsibility of school staff.

Data from both students and staff suggested that the most effective intervention was "the physical presence of a teacher who knew the students and was willing to intervene, coupled with a clear, consistent administrative policy on violence" (p. 34). Expensive security measures (e.g., guards, metal detectors, video cameras) were considered to be ineffective unless integrated into a more comprehensive school response. This study is an excellent example of the use of spatial mapping, in conjunction with interview procedures, as an effective method for exploring predisposing and preventive factors related to school violence.

Elicitation Techniques

In the formative phase of a community-based sexual risk prevention project (Nastasi et al., 1998–1999; Nastasi, Schensul, Ratnayake, & Varjas, 1996; Silva et al., 1997), we used a pilesort technique to elicit definitions of the cultural domains of sexual behaviors and sexual risks from youths ages 17 to 19. Analysis of data from previously conducted in-depth interviews (which included questions about sexual experiences, e.g., in intimate, love, or sexual relationships; Silva et al., 1997) yielded a category of "sexual or intimacy behavior," with 20 terms or descriptors ranging from "holding hands" to "full vaginal penetration." These terms were used in an individually oriented pilesort activity with a sample of 35 older adolescents, ages 17 to 19 (Nastasi et al., 1998–1999). Using the same set of cards, the youths were asked to do three consecutive pilesorts: (a) sort in as many piles as you wish; (b) make two piles—sexual versus nonsexual; and (c) make two piles— safe versus unsafe. The instructions reflect the multiple objectives of the researchers, that is, to gather information about how youths conceptualized distinctions within the domain of sexual or intimacy behaviors (option a) and to force respondents to distinguish terms on a predetermined basis (sex–nonsex and safe–unsafe, options b and c, respectively). Follow-up questions then focused on the individual's rationale for placing terms in respective categories.

Successful conduct of the formative research activities of Phase 5 requires careful framing of research questions, selection of appropriate data sources and data collection methods, and systematic analysis and interpretation of data. It is critical that program planners involve professional researchers (e.g., from the school district, local universities, or community research institutes) in the process of planning and conducting research activities and in training and supervising research staff. Collaboration between intervention and research staff can prove to be mutually beneficial (e.g., for mental health practitioner and university researcher) and strengthen the integration of research and school-based practice.

PHASE 6: CULTURE-SPECIFIC THEORY OR MODEL

The participatory problem-solving and decision-making process described in Phase 3 is applied during this phase to (a) construct a conceptual model that takes into account local culture, (b) identify targets for intervention, and (c) begin to formulate a plan of action. In Exhibit 4.11, we outline the key considerations for Phase 6. Using formative research data collected in Phase 5, participants identify themes relevant to the original theoretical model and constructs, redefine constructs (e.g., stressors, resources, competencies), and revise the initial conceptual model (e.g., add or remove constructs, revise theoretical explanations such as agents and paths of influence) to fit the local culture (e.g., behavioral norms, values, language).

The use of data from multiple sources and methods to guide the generation of local theory is likely to yield both consistencies and discrepancies in definitions of key constructs. The participatory problem-solving process provides a mechanism for addressing discrepancies in data, negotiating resolution of culture conflicts within the target community (e.g., between school and neighborhood behavioral norms, or male and female gender norms), and ensuring that data interpretation accurately reflects stakeholder views (i.e., member checking). Through these activities, program planners can identify gaps in knowledge or discrepancies in data that require additional data collection. Inherent in the ethnographic approach is an iterative process in which researchers return to earlier stages of the data collection–analysis–interpretation process until disconfirming evidence can be incorporated into the explanatory model. This iterative process is likely to continue through the subsequent phases of PCSIM as program design, implementation, and evaluation lead to new questions. For example, data collected during program implementation may lead to refinement or redefinition of

EXHIBIT 4.11
Key Considerations for Phase 6: Culture-Specific Theory or Model

Focus (key questions)—Why?

- What theoretical model best represents the phenomena or problems in the local context?
- What are possible targets for intervention or prevention?
- What are possible actions based on formative data and local theory?

Participants—Who?

- Program planner or planners (researcher, interventionist, consultant)
- Professional(s) with expertise in mental health theory, research, and practice
- Cultural brokers (who can facilitate access and interpret culture)
- Representatives of stakeholder groups

Tasks or Activities—What?

- Review and summarize professional literature on mental health for dissemination to stakeholders
- Prepare formative data and findings for dissemination to stakeholders
- Conduct feedback sessions for the purpose of member checking (verifying data interpretation with representatives of target groups)
- Conduct participatory sessions with partners for the purposes of (a) disseminating and interpreting literature review and formative data, (b) constructing culture-specific theory, and (c) developing action plans

Strategies or Methods—How?

- Review and interpretation of professional literature on children's mental health
- Review and interpretation of formative research findings
- Disseminate and discuss data with representatives of target groups
- Culture-specific theory construction through integration of existing theory and research with formative research findings
- Participatory data-based decision making
- Participatory action planning

Requisite Skills (potential focus for recruitment and training)

- Reviewing and summarizing professional literature on mental health for dissemination to various stakeholder groups
- Translating formative research findings for dissemination to various stakeholder groups
- Data-based decision making and action planning
- Participatory problem-solving skills—communication, negotiation, consensus building
- Group facilitation skills (e.g., engaging participants in idea generation, ensuring equitable participation, guiding group toward consensus)

Challenges

- Communicate findings in acceptable and comprehensible manner to diverse audiences
- Negotiate divergent perspectives among stakeholders to achieve consensus
- Integrating the etic (outsider) perspective of program planners–researchers with emic (insider) perspective of stakeholders or consumers
- Achieve commitment of necessary time and effort from stakeholders
- Overcome existing hierarchical structure or orientation of system to establish equitable partnership roles
- Overcome preference for expert approach to program development

(continued)

EXHIBIT 4.11   *(Continued)*

Opportunities

- Ensure ecological validity and cultural specificity of mental health programs
- Develop model to guide programming that reflects an integrated emic–etic perspective
- Engage in data-based approach to decision making and program planning
- Construct programs tailored to needs and resources of target population or culture
- Foster acceptability and ownership of change efforts
- Build local capacity for culture-specific theory development and action planning

key constructs. Additionally, ongoing data collection can help to ensure that the experiences and interpretations of program participants are addressed.

Illustration 1

In our research in Sri Lanka (the SLMH Project; Nastasi, Varjas, Sarkar, & Jayasena, 1998), formative research influenced our conceptual model in several ways. First, data confirmed alcoholism as a primary stressor for a school-age population. Data collected in Phases 1 and 2 suggested alcoholism as a primary social concern among both adolescents and adults and resulted in the inclusion of alcoholism as a primary stressor in our conceptual model. Second, formative data provided explanations of how psychological stress was engendered. For example, adolescents revealed that stress resulted from parental conflict, domestic violence, shame within the community, and disruption of study time at home. Third, interview data helped us to identify natural sources of emotional support and to understand the conditions under which different resources were enlisted. For example, students identified parents as a preferred resource for dealing with difficulties. When a family problem was the source of stress, however, students sought support from older siblings, peers, or teachers.

Illustration 2

Formative research focused on HIV/AIDS prevention with adolescents in Sri Lanka and the United States provided (a) critical information about the salience of AIDS as an adolescent concern, (b) the cultural scripts surrounding sexual relationships and behaviors (Nastasi et al., 1998–1999), and (c) adolescent youth norms related to sexual practices (J. J. Schensul, 1998–1999). Two key findings had important implications for development of AIDS prevention programs. First, AIDS is not a primary concern of adolescents. Instead, issues such as pregnancy (United States) and virginity (Sri Lanka) are more salient to youths. Second, adolescents or youths engage in unique culturally defined sequences of sexual behaviors, many of which are nonpenetrative. The first finding raised questions about existing AIDS prevention programs that focus primarily on AIDS symptoms, transmission, and prevention strategies. Given the greater concern within the target population for preventing pregnancy or preserving virginity (vs. preventing AIDS), it was important for program developers to broaden the definitions of sexual risks and the focus of the sexual risk prevention programs. In addition, the second finding raised questions about how sex is defined, what abstinence means, and what "not engaging in sex" implies to youths within different cultural contexts. For example, in both settings, researchers identified a number of nonpenetrative sexual practices considered normative (within the respective culture) by youths and found variations in definitions of what constitutes sex for youths. The resulting intervention program in Sri Lanka focused on helping youths to identify type of risk and level of risk for the range of normative "sexual" behaviors. HIV/AIDS became one focus of the intervention. Although HIV/AIDS was the primary concern of funders and researchers, it was clearly a lesser priority for the adolescent–youth population. This work calls attention to the importance of examining the perspective of target individuals as decisions are made about the focus of funding, research, or intervention.

SUMMARY

This chapter addressed the initial research phases of the PCSIM process. Phases 1 through 6 are devoted to developing partnerships, identifying foci for intervention, and constructing a culture-specific conceptual framework to guide mental health programming. The exhibits and illustrations are intended to assist program planners as they initiate entry into systems, form relationships, and gather formative data. The intervention phases (Phases 7–11) described in the next chapter focus on the articulation, delivery, and evaluation of mental health services.

5

PARTICIPATORY CULTURE-SPECIFIC INTERVENTION: PROGRAM (INTERVENTION) PHASES

In this chapter, we describe and illustrate the procedures relevant to the program (intervention) phases, Phases 7 through 11, of the participatory culture-specific intervention model (PCSIM; see Exhibit 3.1 and Figure 3.1, chap. 3, this volume). The structure of this chapter is similar to that for chapter 4. We outline key considerations for each phase in tabular form, provide examples from our work and the work of other researchers and practitioners, and discuss challenges and issues that are likely to confront program planners.

Psychologists, as school-based mental health professionals, are in a key position to provide leadership in developing and implementing comprehensive mental health programs. The scope of such programming, however, precludes solitary efforts. As with the activities of Phases 1 through 6, successful application of PCSIM depends on collaboration among a wide range of stakeholders. The activities of Phases 7 through 11, in particular, require expertise in program design, staff development, and evaluation research. Program planners may need to enlist the help of school- and community-based professionals with expertise in these areas and provide training for nonprofessional stakeholders (e.g., parents, community members).

PHASE 7: PROGRAM DESIGN (PARTICIPATORY GENERATION)

In Phase 7, program planners, working in collaboration with stakeholders, generate a culture-specific mental health promotion program based on the formative research data and culture-specific theory that are the products of Phases 5 and 6, respectively. Formative data from Phase 5 provide the basis for identifying mental health needs of the target population; designing interventions (e.g., strategies and content) or modifying existing programs; developing tools for screening, identification, and evaluation; and identifying necessary and available resources. For example, program planners can use situations described by children to create hypothetical scenarios for teaching coping skills or as an evaluation tool (e.g., self-report or analogue problem-solving scenarios) to assess coping skills.

Phase 7 considerations, outlined in Exhibit 5.1, reflect the complexity of comprehensive program planning. Developing comprehensive programs requires planning for the following: (a) providing a continuum of services, ranging from promotion of mental health for all students to treatment of specific mental health problems of identified students; (b) coordinating and integrating services at building, system, and interagency levels; (c) addressing the various ecological contexts relevant to students (e.g., school, family, peer group, community); (d) designing a program for systematic evaluation of program acceptability, integrity, and evaluation; and (e) addressing individual, contextual, and cultural variations in needs and resources. In addition to these broad issues, specific program features require consideration. These include, but are not limited to, program objectives, intervention strategies and content, screening and identification procedures, staffing and staff training, resource availability and allocation, and evaluation tools. The survey in Appendix 5.1 provides a checklist to guide planning of program specifics.[1]

In this section, we address specific issues in the context of planning for three broad program considerations: (a) continuum of services, (b) service coordination and integration, and (c) family and community involvement. In subsequent phases, we address three additional broad considerations: (d) staff development (Phase 8), (e) program adaptations (Phase 8), and (f) program evaluation (Phase 9).

Continuum of Services

One characteristic of comprehensive school-based mental health programming is the inclusion of a full continuum of services designed to address

---

[1]The survey was designed for a follow-up study of school psychologists' involvement in the design, implementation, and evaluation of mental health programs, funded by the National Association of School Psychologists (Nastasi et al., 2002). Results from the initial study can be found in Nastasi,

the needs of all students, by providing programs to promote mental health, reduce risk for mental health problems, address mental health concerns early, and treat mental illness (USDHHS, 1999). We use a four-level model that encompasses prevention (Level I), risk reduction (Level II), early intervention (Level III), and treatment (Level IV; Meyers & Nastasi, 1998; Nastasi, 1998, 2000). This model is a modification of G. Caplan's (1964) model of primary, secondary, and tertiary levels of prevention programming. Levels I and II correspond to Caplan's primary level, Level III to secondary, and Level IV to tertiary. Consistent with an ecological perspective, interventions at each level target both the individuals and the contexts (e.g., school, family, and neighborhood) that influence the individuals. Achieving a continuum of services requires establishing goals, intervention strategies, identification procedures, staff, and evaluation procedures relevant to each level. In addition, program planners need to establish procedures to ensure the integration and coordination of services across the continuum.

Decisions about the specific elements of a continuum of services are influenced by the formative research and culture-specific conceptual model. Critical to this phase are professionals with expertise in mental health programming and knowledge of evidence-based mental health interventions. The knowledge base relevant to planning a continuum of services is likely to be beyond the expertise of any given mental health professional. Program planners will need to consult with a range of professionals and make use of professional literature to identify previously validated interventions. Selecting evidence-based interventions, however, does not eliminate the need for context-specific program design, adaptation, and evaluation.

Level I: Prevention

School-based prevention programs are directed toward the general population of students within the target system or building. The purpose of Level I programs is the *promotion of mental health* as defined by the U.S. Surgeon General, that is, as "successful performance of mental function, resulting in productive activities, fulfilling relationships with other people, and the ability to adapt to change and to cope with adversity" (USDHHS, 1999, p. 8). School-based mental health promotion encompasses efforts to foster culturally valued competencies (e.g., cognitive–academic, social–emotional, behavioral), developmentally appropriate and socially valid relationship skills (e.g., communication, negotiation, peaceful conflict resolution), and culturally relevant coping skills (e.g., personal and interpersonal

Varjas, Bernstein, and Pluymert (1998a, 1998b). This version of the survey (Appendix 5.1) is an abbreviated form of that used in the original study and is reprinted with permission from the National Association of School Psychologists.

EXHIBIT 5.1
Key Considerations for Phase 7: Program Design
(Participatory Generation)

Focus (key questions)—Why?

- What are the goals and objectives of programming (based on formative research and culture-specific theory)?
- What levels of the intervention continuum (prevention to treatment) are included?
- What prevention or intervention strategies and content are consistent with goals and objectives?
- How do we integrate proposed program efforts with existing programs in school and community; that is, how do we best achieve integration and coordination of services?
- How do we link assessment–evaluation and intervention as a seamless process?
- How do we address the individual and contextual diversity within the system?
- What are the necessary staff qualifications? How do we secure staff involvement? How do we make the best use of existing staff resources within school and community?
- What procedures are necessary to provide consultation, support, and training for staff?
- What procedures are necessary for identifying participants, obtaining consent, and determining the nature and scope of intervention–treatment?
- What are relevant forms of family involvement? How do we secure family involvement?
- How do we address legal and ethical issues relevant to mental health intervention within schools?
- What resources are necessary for program implementation and evaluation? What resources are available within the school and community? How do we gain access to available resources? How do we secure additional required resources?
- How do we ensure implementation of program activities?
- How do we ensure program sustainability and institutional or community capacity building?
- What structure and process are necessary to ensure that program goals are achieved?
- What structure and process are necessary to ensure participation of stakeholders?

Participants—Who?

- Program planner or planners (researcher, interventionist, consultant)
- Professionals with expertise in mental health program design, systems change, and organizational consultation
- Professionals with expertise in securing funds
- Professionals and paraprofessionals with expertise in mental health prevention or intervention
- Cultural brokers (who can facilitate access and interpret culture)
- Staff from school departments and community agencies who provide relevant services
- Representatives of stakeholder groups (including students, parents, administrators, teachers, and other school personnel)

Tasks or Activities—What?

- Identify program goals and objectives
- Select or develop program components and intervention strategies
- Identify staff needs, secure staff, and provide necessary training
- Secure funding and other necessary resources
- Establish procedures for screening, identifying, and providing services to students

(continued)

EXHIBIT 5.1 *(Continued)*

- Establish procedures for coordination of services and case management
- Establish infrastructure and process for program implementation, management, monitoring, and evaluation
- Establish participatory process for involving stakeholders
- Identify roles and responsibilities of partners
- Establish system for communication among school staff, community staff, and other stakeholders
- Convene planning team with representatives of stakeholder groups
- Facilitate participatory planning process

Strategies or Methods—How?

- Program development and evaluation
- Intervention design
- Staff development
- Team process or collaborative problem solving
- Organizational consultation

Requisite Skills (potential focus for recruitment and training)

- Program development and evaluation
- Systems change and organizational consultation
- Staff development
- Professional expertise relevant to selected programs and intervention and evaluation strategies
- Program administration, management, and coordination
- Fiscal and other resource management
- Interagency collaboration
- Participatory problem-solving skills—communication, negotiation, consensus building
- Group facilitation skills (e.g., engaging participants in idea generation, ensuring equitable participation, guiding group toward consensus)

Challenges

- Overcome resistance to change within existing organizations or systems
- Overcome territorial boundaries across different groups of professionals
- Identify or create appropriate evidence-based programs
- Achieve commitment of necessary time and effort from stakeholders
- Secure necessary resources
- Negotiate across policy and procedural variations of participating agencies, organizations, departments
- Overcome existing hierarchical structure or orientation of system to establish equitable partnership roles

Opportunities

- Ensure ecological validity and cultural specificity of mental health programs
- Promote stakeholder involvement, ownership, and empowerment
- Establish sustainable and institutionalized process for participatory program development
- Build local capacity for designing comprehensive and culturally specific mental health programs
- Develop mental health programming skills among professionals and paraprofessionals
- Involve families and community members and agencies in mental health programming
- Achieve intra- and interagency integration and coordination of services (coordinated system of mental health care)

problem solving). Furthermore, Level I programs are directed toward the prevention of social morbidities described in chapter 1, such as violence, drug abuse and related injuries, sexual risks and sexually transmitted diseases, suicide, homelessness, and school dropout. Comprehensive mental health promotion covers social, emotional, behavioral, cognitive, and academic aspects of individual functioning, and thus requires integration rather than separation of cognitive–academic and social–emotional–behavioral goals within educational programs. Examples of Level I school-based programs include the following: (a) *Everybody's Different*, a classroom-based education program to prevent eating disorders among adolescents (O'Dea & Abraham, 2000); (b) *Stand Together Against Negative Decisions (STAND)*, a peer education training program to promote abstinence and reduce sexual risk among adolescents (originally implemented at the community level and then applied and tested in schools; M. U. Smith & DiClemente, 2000); (c) *Life Skills Training (LST)*, a curriculum-based substance abuse prevention program for students in Grades 7 to 9 (Botvin, Baker, Dusenbury, Botvin, & Diaz, 1995; Botvin, Baker, Dusenbury, Tortu, & Botvin, 1990; Botvin, Schinke, Epstein, Diaz, & Botvin, 1995); (d) *I Can Problem Solve (ICPS)*, a classroom-based (teacher-implemented) program to develop interpersonal problem-solving skills in children ages 4 to 12 (preschool and elementary grade level programs; Shure, 1996); and (e) *Child Development Project*, a comprehensive building-level program to foster prosocial school norms and individual prosocial development (Battistich, Schaps, Watson, & Solomon, 1996; Battistich, Solomon, Watson, Solomon, & Schaps, 1989).

To ensure availability to all students, Level I activities are an integral part of schoolwide and classroomwide programs. At the schoolwide level, prevention goals are reflected throughout the school culture, for example, in discipline policies and procedures, adult–student and administrator–staff relationships, schoolwide activities, and the school mission. Mental health promotion and risk prevention programs are part of the classroom curriculum across all grade levels. The curriculum across classrooms and grade levels reflects an overarching scope and sequence consistent with schoolwide or districtwide mental health goals. School policies and behavioral norms are consistent with the underlying concepts of classroom-based mental health programs. For example, if students are taught certain strategies for resolving interpersonal conflicts, those strategies are used throughout the school (in classrooms, cafeteria, assemblies, playground, and field trips) by staff as well as students. Such comprehensive implementation requires commitment and skill development for all staff, including administrators, teachers, mental health and health professionals, security officers, support staff, and volunteer staff. In addition, effective and sustained implementation requires ongoing support and consultation by mental health staff, an issue we discuss in Phase 8.

Level II: Risk Reduction

Level II programming efforts are directed to those students who are at high risk for developing mental health problems or mental illness (see definitions in Exhibit 1.1, chap. 1, this volume) as a result of individual or cultural vulnerabilities. Examples of Level II school-based programs include the following: (a) *Children of Divorce Intervention Project (CODIP)*, for elementary school age children, to promote adjustment to parental divorce (Pedro-Carroll, 1997); (b) *Project ACHIEVE*, a comprehensive building-level program targeted at (preschool–elementary) schools serving at-risk populations based on social–cultural indicators (e.g., racial–ethnic minority, low socioeconomic status; Knoff & Batsche, 1995); and (c) *crisis intervention programs* to organize system-level response, manage crises, and prevent or reduce posttraumatic stress disorder resulting from school or community disasters or trauma (e.g., natural disaster, incidents of violence, or death; Klingman, 1996; Pitcher & Poland, 1992).

The purpose of Level II activities is to provide more intensive intervention directed toward the development of culturally valued competencies, interpersonal skills, and coping skills. In addition, intervention efforts are directed toward bolstering social–cultural supports or resources as well as individual or personal resources. Culture-specific vulnerabilities are identified through formative research and development of culture-specific theory in Phases 5 and 6. For example, in our work in Sri Lanka (Nastasi, Varjas, Sarkar, & Jayasena, 1998), we identified parental alcoholism as a risk factor for childhood stress and adjustment difficulties in both extant literature and formative research findings and included it in our culture-specific model as a social–cultural stressor and potential personal vulnerability factor. In other settings, early exposure to domestic or community violence, parental divorce, or poverty might be identified as culture-specific risk factors. Furthermore, individual factors such as learning problems, poor school attendance, or truancy might be identified as risk factors (personal vulnerabilities) for social morbidities such as school dropout, delinquency, or drug abuse. Although extant research literature provides potential indicators of risk for mental health problems or illness, it is critical that program planners provide culture-specific evidence through formative research.

The use of systemwide screening procedures can facilitate identification of at-risk students (e.g., children of alcoholics; Nastasi, 1995; depression, W. R. Reynolds, 1986; anxiety, Laurent, Hadler, & Stark, 1994). In addition, Level I activities provide a context for identifying those at high risk for mental health problems. For example, screening activities can be integrated into classroom-based curriculum, or teachers can be encouraged to pay close attention to student comments and consult with or make referrals to mental health professionals when concerns arise. Mental health professionals (e.g., school psychologists) can play an important role in development or identification of screening instruments, training of teachers in early identification, and establishing effective referral procedures.

Level II interventions also require enlisting mental health professionals (from within the school or larger community) who have expertise in addressing the target risk factors. Alternatively, mental health professionals train paraprofessionals to provide direct services (e.g., Cowen et al., 1996). This alternative, however, necessitates ongoing consultation and support from mental health professionals.

Level III: Early Intervention

Early intervention efforts represent even more intensive services directed to students who are either at risk or currently experiencing mild mental health problems or adjustment difficulties. The goals of Level III are to provide intervention to address current mental health problems, reduce the risk of exacerbation of problems, and prevent (diagnosable) mental illness. These efforts are directed at an even smaller proportion of the school population and require the expertise of mental health professionals or experienced paraprofessionals with supervision and support by mental health staff. Early intervention is provided to students individually or in small groups and focuses on specific problems that students are experiencing as well as skills or competencies for reducing the risk of more serious problems. In contrast to Level I and Level II interventions, which are characterized as education and skill building, Level III interventions take the form of counseling or therapy.

Formative research findings can provide information about the needs and resources relevant to mental health problems within the target population, and thus facilitate planning efforts. In addition, specific concerns may arise during the implementation of Level I and Level II activities. Given the potential variation in mental health problems within a given population, program planners may need to enlist the expertise of mental health professionals working in the community. Furthermore, Level III activities encompass early intervention for problems related to both psychiatric disorders (e.g., depression) and social morbidities (substance abuse), thus extending the scope of necessary professional expertise.

Examples of Level III school-based programs include the following: (a) *Family and Schools Together (FAST)*, designed to strengthen families (single parent, living in poverty, racial minority) of high-risk youths (elementary and middle school; scoring as at-risk on a teacher rating of behavior) and reduce familial stress and the child's risk of school failure and substance abuse (McDonald & Sayger, 1998); and (b) *combined parent and school early intervention programs for preschool or kindergarten-age boys* exhibiting disruptive behavior, to facilitate school adjustment and reduce the risk of later school difficulties (Barkley et al., 2000; Tremblay, Pagani-Kurtz, Masse, Vitaro, & Pihl, 1995). Also illustrative are three group-based intervention programs for reducing the risk of internalizing disorders or difficulties: (a) *Personal Growth Class (PGC)*, to facilitate social support networks and reduce suicidal risk (Eggert et al., 1995); (b) *Coping With Stress Course*, to prevent unipolar depressive disorders (Clarke et al., 1995); and (c) *Coping Koala*, to prevent anxiety disorders (Dadds et al., 1999). All three programs were implemented in the school setting and used multistage screening to identify adolescents at risk and currently experiencing at least mild difficulties but not yet meeting diagnostic criteria for the target difficulty or disorder.

Identification of candidates for early intervention can take several forms. Students can self-identify or be referred by parents, teachers, or other school personnel on the basis of symptoms exhibited in the normal course of daily activities. Mental health professionals can facilitate referrals by developing lists of symptoms and educational venues (written materials, presentations, workshops) for parents and school personnel. Level I programs can include information about mental health problems (i.e., signs, symptoms, prevalence, treatment) and encourage students to contact school-based mental health professionals with concerns. Mental health professionals can offer programs specifically geared toward problems identified during formative data collection (e.g., significant proportion of students expressing social anxiety).

Students also can be identified with a systematic multistage screening procedure in which progressively more intensive assessment is used on fewer and fewer students (suicide, Eggert et al., 1995; anxiety, Laurent et al., 1994; depression, W. R. Reynolds, 1986). For example, a general self-report screening measure is used systemwide to identify students who are experiencing symptoms of depression or anxiety. Using a normative cutoff point (based on national or local norms), mental health professionals can identify a smaller sample of students for a second screening. Those who meet the cutoff criteria a second time are identified for more in-depth multimethod, multisource evaluation (e.g., with a self-report diagnostic measure, semistructured diagnostic interview, parent and teacher reports, and classroom observations). Those who meet the criteria for mild depression or anxiety are then selected for participation in a risk reduction intervention that is focused, for example, on relieving depression or anxiety, teaching cognitive coping strategies, and monitoring symptoms.

Level IV: Treatment

Level IV efforts are designed for the select proportion of students who are diagnosed with psychiatric disorders or exhibit moderate to severe levels of social morbidities (e.g., suicidal or homicidal behavior) and who require intensive treatment by credentialed medical or mental health professionals. The students who warrant Level IV services may qualify for special education services, but this is not necessarily the case. Care can take the form of individual or group psychotherapy, pharmacological treatment, or both and may involve the student as well as family members. Examples of school-based Level IV programs include the following: (a) services provided through *school-based mental health or health clinics* (Armbruster & Litchman, 1999; Flaherty & Weist, 1999; Hannah & Nichol, 1996; Ring-Kurtz et al., 1995; Weist, Paskewitz, Warner, & Flaherty, 1996); (b) *systems of care* that involve school–community collaboration (Attkisson et al., 1995; Attkisson et al., 1997; Jordan, 1996); and (c) *individually oriented direct or indirect interventions* targeting students with specific disorders, such as attention deficit hyperactivity disorder (DuPaul & Eckert, 1997; Shapiro & DuPaul, 1996; Sheridan, Dee, Morgan, McCormick, & Walker, 1996).

With the exception of those with school-based or school-linked clinics, schools are typically ill-equipped to provide Level IV services that go beyond academic intervention. Thus, students with moderate to severe mental health difficulties are likely to require referral to outpatient or inpatient community-based mental health facilities. School-based mental health professionals (e.g., school psychologists) can play an important liaison role in Level IV service provision, for example, making initial referrals, facilitating communication with community agencies, and planning for students' transition back to school following inpatient (residential) treatment. In addition, school-based mental health professionals can provide education to school staff, parents, and students about psychiatric disorders and social morbidities (e.g., warning signs, symptoms, resources, treatment); participate in identification and diagnosis of students; and provide consultation to teachers about classroom-based interventions to facilitate adjustment of students with moderate to severe difficulties.

Service Coordination and Integration

The coordination and integration of services embodied in the four-level continuum are critical to effective implementation and program success, yet present a major challenge to program planners and administrators. Management of the host of services and staff is complicated further by the participation of professionals from different departments within the school system and from different agencies outside of the school system. In addition, mental health needs and programming are not necessarily the primary concern of schools and are often secondary to academic priorities. Furthermore, comprehensive service provision involves collaboration across several professional disciplines, with different theoretical and empirical foundations, techniques, ethical guidelines, and priorities. Indeed, the complex nature of mental health (as defined in chap. 1, this volume) necessitates collaboration among professionals from disciplines such as psychology, medicine, public health, social work, anthropology, sociology, and criminology. The integration of mental health service in schools extends the interdisciplinary network to include other professionals such as educators, language specialists, and systems specialists. The network of organizations is likely to include schools, hospitals, health and mental health clinics, child protection agencies, police departments, and, in some instances, universities and other research institutions. Finally, the comprehensive approach involves the participation of nonprofessional or paraprofessional stakeholders such as family and community members. Bringing together the various disciplines, stakeholders, and services can be a daunting task.

The importance of service coordination and integration is evident in recent efforts to address school violence. For example, in response to school shootings that occurred in the United States in the 1990s, the U.S. Secret Service and U.S. Department of Education (2002) collaborated in the study of school shootings and development of guidelines for managing threatening situations and promoting safe schools. The guidelines call for establishing school-based threat assessment teams that include representatives of staff from the school district and local law enforcement and mental health agencies. The threat assessment team is charged with the responsibility of developing policies and procedures for identifying, assessing, and managing threatening situations. In addition, the team makes recommendations for program implementation, staff training, monitoring and evaluation, and necessary modifications.

How Does One Achieve Effective Service Coordination and Integration?

We draw on our own professional experiences and knowledge for insights, recommendations, and cautions (see Exhibit 5.2). It is probable that the most critical component of effective coordination and integration is communication. The participatory problem-solving process described in chapter 4 is as applicable to sustaining ongoing communication as it is to establishing partnerships and early decision making. The size of the system may necessitate multiple teams operating within buildings, across the school system, and across agencies. The complexity of the school system and interorganizational network determines the complexity of the team process. To illustrate, we use a prototypical system that represents urban school systems and communities in the United States.

Illustration

The system has approximately 100 schools, including elementary, middle, junior high, high school, and alternative schools. Administrators at the

EXHIBIT 5.2
Coordination and Integration of Comprehensive Services:
Insights, Recommendations, and Cautions

Insights

- Regular and open communication is essential.
- Respect for different perspectives is critical to finding common ground.
- Everyone at the table has something valuable to offer to the process.
- Commitment to a common goal is the place to start and return to throughout the process.
- There is no substitute for one-to-one contact on a regular basis.
- Day-to-day problem solving is a necessity.
- Flexibility is paramount.
- As with any team, both group responsibility and individual accountability are necessary.
- Many factors, not always predictable, influence success. The key is finding ways to capitalize on and increase facilitators and circumvent or remove inhibitors.
- Maintaining the sense of accomplishment, self-esteem, and self-efficacy of all the players (stakeholders, staff, students) is as important as implementing program activities with integrity.
- The mental health of the staff is as critical as the mental health of the students.
- More is not necessarily better: A conglomeration of disconnected programs not only can be a waste of resources, but also may negate our best efforts.
- Without evaluation, there is no assurance of program effectiveness.
- A well-coordinated, integrated system takes time to develop and requires continuous maintenance.
- Change takes time and effort, much more than we ever anticipate.

Recommendations

- Bring key players together on a regular basis.
- Make sure the communication network is iterative and includes those on the front line.
- Institute a central position or location (office, person, team) for the flow of information and the coordination of programs and activities. Depending on the size of the system and scope of services, such a position may be necessary in each building as well as the central office.
- Establish clear goals and objectives that are comprehensible and agreeable to all stakeholders.
- Weigh the value of each program or intervention against the goals of comprehensive mental health service delivery.
- Make sure staff members from different programs communicate with each other.
- Establish and monitor a system of accountability.
- Institute an evaluation program to guide decision making about continuation and alterations in programming.
- Make the goals and objectives of comprehensive service delivery clear to all stakeholders.
- Use goals and objectives as the benchmarks for decision making.
- Monitor the well-being of stakeholders (students, staff, community members, administrators), and plan ways to bolster the self-esteem, self-efficacy, and sense of accomplishment of all stakeholders.
- Develop a plan for dealing with day-to-day as well as major crises.

Cautions

- Avoid bringing in new services or programs unless they meet overall goals and objectives.

(continued)

EXHIBIT 5.2   *(Continued)*

- Avoid operating in a crisis mode.
- Seek out information before making decisions.
- Initial agreement does not necessarily mean continual agreement. Likewise, initial disagreement does not mean agreement can never occur.
- Service coordination and integration is a process—be patient.
- Avoid lapsing into a hierarchical mode. Instead bring the players back to the table.
- There is no substitute for open and regular communication.
- No one gets their way all the time—collaboration requires compromise.
- Avoid the tendency to provide minimal training and expect staff to become experts overnight.
- Investigate lapses in communication or responsibilities. The problem is not always apparent.

system's level include the superintendent, several assistant superintendents, and department heads (e.g., math, science, health, evaluation, truancy, transportation). At the building level, depending on the size of the school, the staff includes principal, assistant principal(s), regular and special education teachers, psychologists, nurses, social workers, counselors, reading specialists, language therapists, teaching assistants, police or security officers, clerical staff, custodial staff, and other support staff. In addition, a building may include tutors, volunteers, and a host of paraprofessionals, parents, or community members who assist with special activities or daily operation of the school. In some buildings, school-based health clinics have been established to provide health and mental health care to students and are staffed with school and community agency employees.

Like many school systems, the district has responded to national and state initiatives for addressing violence, school safety, drug education, reproductive health and AIDS education, social skills, and conflict resolution. Each year the district adds new programs and removes others. Programs are replaced when initiatives or funding priorities change, or in response to local crises. In addition to the health, safety, and mental health initiatives, the district is continually responding to new initiatives to enhance and monitor academic achievement (e.g., bringing in new curricula, establishing new testing programs). Each of these initiatives brings with it demands for staff development, material and personnel resources, funding, and revisiting or changing priorities.

Furthermore, the schools are located in communities with a host of health and social service agencies that provide services to the staff, students, and families within the district or have the potential to contribute to a comprehensive system of mental health care. Such agencies might include hospitals, health and mental health clinics, child protection agency, police department, judicial system, private educational institutions, research agencies, and universities. These agencies employ a range of professionals and paraprofessionals with expertise relevant to promoting the mental health and safety of students, and who can assist in program design, implementation, and evaluation. Furthermore, there are government and private sources of funding at local, state, and national levels to support school-based mental health efforts.

Let us assume that this school system has engaged in the PCSIM process through Phase 6. There is agreement among stakeholders to design a comprehensive school-based mental health promotion program that would provide the continuum of services delivered by a network of professionals from the school system and partner mental health and social service agencies. The question is not one of commitment—partners are in consensus about the needs, goals, and scope of the program. The question is not about the availability of resources or recognition of need for coordinated, integrated services for students. The question is, *What will it take to establish and maintain well-coordinated, integrated comprehensive mental health services for students in the school district?* We address this question at multiple levels, beginning at the district level.

Program planners help to establish a *district-level interagency mental health team,* which includes representatives of administrative, teaching, and mental health personnel from the school district and from the partner agencies. The purpose of this team is to design a structure and process for ensuring regular and open communication across agencies and within the district. The team decides first to gather information about the stakeholders, existing programs, and resources at the district, school building, and agency levels. The team then uses the information to make decisions about the structure and process for service coordination and integration. Their recommendations follow.

1. The district-level mental health team would be responsible for system-level and interagency oversight. Responsibilities would include the following: (a) meeting on a regular basis; (b) reviewing all proposals within the district for new or revised mental health intervention programs to ensure consistency with overall goals; (c) ensuring that each program includes an evaluation plan and a plan for integration with existing programs; (d) calling for periodic reports on all programs; (e) using evaluation data to monitor program acceptability, integrity, effectiveness, and integration; (f) monitoring district needs related to mental health programming; (g) making data-based recommendations for establishing new programs and continuing, combining, or terminating existing programs; and (h) addressing discrepancies across agencies that inhibit infor-

mation sharing and service coordination (e.g., issues related to confidentiality of information, overlap of services by different providers, territorial issues among professionals).

2. The district-level mental health team would expand its membership to include representatives of other stakeholders groups, such as students, parents, community members, and legislators. In addition, the team will monitor its membership to ensure that all relevant stakeholder groups are included.

3. Each building would establish a mental health team with representation of the stakeholder groups for that building, including school system personnel, partner agency personnel, students, parents, and community members. The responsibilities and activities of the building-level team would match those of the district-level team. For example, the building-level team would be responsible for reviewing program proposals for the building, monitoring program evaluation and integration, and making data-based decisions. In addition, they would report to the district-level team on an ongoing basis. Each building-level team also would have representation on the district-level team.

4. All teams would receive training and follow-up consultation on the participatory problem-solving and decision-making process and engage in ongoing self-evaluation of the team process.

5. The district-level team, with input from building-level teams, would develop a plan for resolving conflicts between district-level and building-level priorities, in a manner that preserves the participatory process.

6. All personnel working within the school buildings (administrative, teaching, support) would receive ongoing training on collaboration and any buildingwide initiatives (e.g., disciplinary plans, conflict resolution strategies).

Family and Community Involvement

Partnership in comprehensive mental health promotion extends to all stakeholders with vested interests or resources. These include family and community members. As we have noted, program planners are encouraged to involve families and community members as partners in the PCSIM process. In the past decade, much has been written about the need for parental involvement and about ways to facilitate such involvement (e.g., Albee & Canetto, 1996; Christenson & Buerkle, 1999; Christenson & Conoley, 1992; Heflinger & Bickman, 1996; Sheridan, Dee, Morgan, McCormick, & Walker, 1996; Sheridan, Kratochwill, & Bergan, 1996). In the next section, we identify several critical considerations and provide suggestions for facilitating involvement of families and community members.

Considerations for Facilitating Involvement

First, parents and community members are likely to be the most disenfranchised stakeholder groups and the least well prepared to engage in a participatory process with school and agency administrators and staff. They do not necessarily have the background experience and knowledge that mental health and educational professionals bring to the table. Their experiences with participating schools and agencies have not necessarily been positive, nor have they necessarily participated as equals with school and agency staff. Furthermore, there are likely to be cultural conflicts between the values, beliefs, ideas, norms, language, and expectations of school or agency personnel and family or community members. Thus, it is the responsibility of school and agency personnel to create a climate that is welcoming to families and community members; to show them respect, without condescension; to listen to and value their contributions; and to include them as equal partners.

Second, parents and community members, like other stakeholders, need opportunities for skill development to participate effectively in the PCSIM process. Nonprofessionals can learn to design and conduct research that leads to action and change (J. J. Schensul, 1998, 1998–1999). Indeed, action research models were initially developed for the purposes of facilitating social change and empowering community members (Kemmis & McTaggart, 2000). Teaching community members to engage in research and data-based decision making has the short-term benefit of enhancing involvement and commitment and the long-term benefit of capacity building. The full involvement of community members as partners in the research and intervention process is dependent on the abilities of program planners and other professional stakeholders to provide skill development and to translate their professional expertise and knowledge into the language of the lay community.

Third, parents and community members have information and perspectives that can enhance the professionals' perspectives and practice. Program planners and professional stakeholders depend on parents, community members, and students to provide the culture specificity that is central to PCSIM. They are the experts on their own culture, and we as researchers and professionals have much to learn from them. An ethnographic perspective is invaluable as we attempt to engage parents and community members in the participatory process. The goal of the ethnographer is to learn about the culture of a group or community or society from the perspective of its members. The ethnographer's role is that of learner, with the community members as their teachers. Successful ethnographic work depends on the researcher's ability to listen, observe, and be open to ideas, customs, and ways of living that may be very different from his or her own. This openness to learning from others is critical to engaging in a truly participatory process and to ensuring culture specificity of the programs we create.

As with other aspects of the PCSIM process, involving parents and community members requires continual attention and monitoring. With consistent effort to involve parents and community members in a meaningful way, they can become productive and valuable partners in creating and sustaining mental health programs for children and adolescents. In the next section, we provide two examples of successful efforts to engage parents and community members in school-based change efforts.

Illustration

The first example comes from the efforts to integrate child psychiatry and education that began in New Haven, Connecticut, in the 1960s (Comer, Haynes, Joyner, & Ben-Avie, 1996). The Social Development Program (SDP), initiated by James Comer, involves parents, teachers, and administrators in a participatory process for planning, implementing, and evaluating comprehensive school plans that address students' social and academic needs. *Parent teams* are designed to engage parents in school planning (as representatives on building-level teams) and teaching and support activities (e.g., assisting in classroom or school library), and to foster home–school collaboration and parental empowerment. Since its inception, the SDP has been implemented in several cities across the United States. (For additional information, readers are encouraged to consult the numerous publications by Comer and his colleagues.)

The second example is drawn from recent work of Stephen Leff in Philadelphia schools (Leff, 2001). Using a participatory approach, Leff successfully engaged paraprofessional partners (parents and other community members) as both interventionists (as playground monitors) and researchers (collecting observational data) in a program to improve students' playground behavior and reduce aggression. This program holds great promise as a model for involving community members in school interventions.

The activities of Phase 7 are focused on designing comprehensive programs based on information gathered in the first six phases and are dependent on the relationships among partners. The process of design does not end as we move to Phase 8. Indeed, the iterative process requires continual return to the considerations of Phase 7. The seamless process inherent in PCSIM makes it difficult to clearly demarcate its phases. In the next section, we address program implementation. We include program adaptations and staff development in Phase 8, although plans for these components must begin in Phase 7 as program planners design the intervention(s).

PHASE 8: PROGRAM IMPLEMENTATION
(NATURAL ADAPTATION)

The most apparent goal of Phase 8 is to carry out the intervention designed in Phase 7. As suggested by the list of considerations for this phase (see Exhibit 5.3), realizing the intervention is a complex task. At a minimum, program implementation involves securing resources, training staff, producing intervention manuals, identifying participants, instituting evaluation activities, and administering project activities. In addition, program implementation within PCSIM necessitates setting up, facilitating, and monitoring a structure and process for participatory decision making. Also inherent in PCSIM is the process of *natural adaptation*, that is, the modification of the predesigned program to match the resources and needs of participants in the natural setting (Nastasi, Varjas, Schensul, et al., 2000). Necessary to the adaptation process is documentation of program implementation as the basis for decision making and for ensuring program integrity. Integrity in this case refers to maintaining the essential or core features of the intervention. Furthermore, maintaining stakeholder involvement, ownership, and empowerment is necessary for successful implementation, sustainability, and institutionalization.

Program Adaptations

The concept of natural adaptation within PCSIM stands in contrast to traditional notions of strict adherence to intervention protocols as necessary for intervention integrity. Adaptation to individual and contextual variation, however, does not imply dispensing with integrity. Instead, the goal is to maintain integrity (i.e., that which is essential for achieving intended outcomes) while permitting modifications that are necessary for applying the intervention successfully in a given context (and across multiple, varied contexts). Thus, adaptation provides flexibility without sacrificing rigor.

Considerations for Achieving Adaptation

Critical to the adaptation process is data-based decision making, which depends on systematic in-depth documentation of the individual and contextual variations that necessitate modifications. The capacity for making informed decisions about modifications depends on delineation of essential (core) versus nonessential (variable) components of the intervention. The delineation of essential and nonessential components requires research to establish the links between intervention components and outcomes. Thus, evaluation research (Phase 9) becomes the basis for decision making.

EXHIBIT 5.3
Key Considerations for Phase 8: Program Implementation
(Natural Adaptation)

Focus (key questions)—Why?

- What adjustments are necessary in the planned intervention to ensure ecological fit?
- How can the program be adapted to specific contexts and participants without violating intervention integrity?
- What are the core (essential) program elements, that is, those that are necessary for program effectiveness?
- What are the flexible (nonessential) program elements, that is, those that can be adapted without impeding program effectiveness?
- What factors facilitate and inhibit implementation?
- What is an effective process for conducting adaptation?
- How do we ensure program acceptability and integrity?
- How do we promote stakeholder involvement, ownership, and empowerment?
- What procedures can we put in place to promote sustainability, institutionalization, and capacity building?
- How do we best involve stakeholders in a participatory process of data-based decision making?

Participants—Who?

- Program planner or planners (researcher, interventionist, consultant)
- Professionals with expertise in mental health program design, implementation, and evaluation; staff development; program coordination and management; and systems change, organizational consultation, and capacity building
- Professionals and paraprofessionals with expertise in mental health prevention or intervention, particularly with skills related to implementing and evaluating program activities
- Cultural brokers (who can facilitate access and interpret culture)
- Staff from school departments and community agencies who provide relevant services
- Representatives of stakeholder groups (including students, parents, administrators, teachers, and other school personnel)

Tasks or Activities—What?

- Educate or train professional and paraprofessional staff
- Provide ongoing staff consultation and support
- Identify program recipients
- Obtain necessary informed consent
- Access necessary resources
- Establish process for program administration, management, and monitoring
- Prepare and distribute program materials
- Schedule program implementation
- Coordinate services
- Make program adaptations
- Institute program evaluation activities
- Document program implementation
- Establish a process and structure for participatory decision making
- Implement participatory decision-making process

(continued)

EXHIBIT 5.3   *(Continued)*

Strategies or Methods—How?

- Documentation of program implementation using combination of qualitative and quantitative methods (see Phase 9)
- Systematic monitoring and feedback process to facilitate program adaptation and staff development
- Participatory consultation approach to staff development and support
- Participatory problem-solving process for data-based decision making
- Facilitation of participatory process

Requisite Skills (potential focus for recruitment and training)

- Program development and adaptation
- Skills relevant to particular intervention strategies
- Staff development and consultation
- Program administration and management
- Expertise in mixed-method program evaluation—data collection, analysis, interpretation, dissemination
- Participatory problem-solving skills—communication, negotiation, consensus building
- Group facilitation skills (e.g., engaging participants in idea generation, ensuring equitable participation, guiding group toward consensus)
- Service integration and coordination (within and across agencies)
- Case management
- Organizational consultation or systems change
- Capacity building

Challenges

- Maintain program acceptability, involvement, and commitment
- Maintain program integrity
- Engage in day-to-day project management and problem solving
- Facilitate communication and collaboration across diverse stakeholders
- Overcome territorial boundaries across different groups of professionals and agencies
- Overcome resistance to change within existing organizations–systems
- Secure commitment to ongoing evaluation (monitoring of implementation)
- Identify and address barriers to successful implementation
- Achieve commitment of necessary time and effort from stakeholders
- Address conflicts for time and resources with other school programs or efforts
- Balance mental health and academic priorities within school system or building
- Respond to crises without interfering with ongoing efforts

Opportunities

- Ensure ecological validity and cultural specificity of mental health programs
- Achieve natural adaptation of planned program to needs and demands of target contexts and participants
- Contribute to knowledge about deployment of evidence-based interventions in real-life settings
- Foster sustainability and institutionalization of mental health programs
- Establish system for integration of intervention and evaluation (accountability, monitoring, program evaluation)
- Establish sustainable system for data-based decision making
- Establish process for participatory decision making
- Build organizational or community capacity
- Enhance attention and commitment to mental health needs of students
- Achieve service coordination at intra- and interagency levels

The potentially infinite range of variations across students, teachers, and classrooms necessitates replication of the adaptation process with each implementation. One aim of capacity building (Phase 10) is to ensure that stakeholders have the skills to repeat the adaptation process in the absence of program planners. In addition, the adaptation process provides a mechanism for translation or deployment (Phase 11) of science-based interventions to real-life settings. Furthermore, replication of the intervention-research process across a wide range of students, teachers, and classrooms contributes to an empirical foundation for informed decision making and advances the knowledge base of individual practitioners and the field of psychology, thus completing the PCSIM cycle.

Achieving adaptation requires recycling through the action-research process (see Figure 2.3, chap. 2, this volume) during implementation. From the initiation of the intervention designed in Phase 7, program evaluators (a) collect data about participant response to intervention strategies and content (intervention acceptability; e.g., through observation and interview with teachers–therapists and students), (b) document intervention sessions (intervention integrity; e.g., through observation, therapist–teacher logs), and (c) evaluate impact of intervention activities (intervention outcome; e.g., observation, self-reports, or informant reports). Data collection continues throughout implementation on a predetermined continual or periodic basis (e.g., weekly, biweekly). Also on a periodic basis, data are prepared for dissemination to program planners and stakeholders and become the basis for their decision making about modifications. For example, planners and evaluators might meet on a weekly basis with teachers (individually or in groups) who are implementing a behavior change program in the classroom. At these meetings, the team (planner, evaluator, teachers) reviews and interprets the data with regard to intervention acceptability, integrity, progress toward goals (impact), and links between process and outcome; identifies potential targets for modification; and develops plans for modification (i.e., retaining what works and changing what is not working). Modifications can involve content or strategy change at the classroom or individual level, additional staff development or training for teachers, or both. The focus throughout these data review and decision-making sessions is to maximize both ecological fit and program effectiveness.

Illustration

We draw from our own experiences in the United States[2] and abroad (Nastasi, Varjas, Bernstein, & Jayasena, 2000) working with teachers who

[2] A 4½-year intervention research project, "Building Preventive Group Norms in Urban Middle Schools," funded by the National Institute on Drug Abuse, National Institutes of Health (Grant No.

are responsible for implementing classroom-based mental health promotion or health risk (drugs, sexual) prevention programs. Teacher requests (based on identified and documented difficulties) for modifications can range from altering materials for student reading level (e.g., in inclusion classroom) or language differences (e.g., in bilingual classroom) to altering core components of the intervention (e.g., disband with group work in a program based on student collaboration).

In the first instance (altering materials), teacher requests are relatively easy to accommodate. Program planners work with the teachers to rewrite materials in simpler language or translate to students' primary language. In addition, the bilingual teacher may want to use program activities to enhance students' language skills, in which case materials are prepared in both the primary language and English and the teacher integrates vocabulary-building activities into the mental health or health risk curriculum. The decisions to make these changes result from teacher–program planner discussions following data collection. In addition, program evaluators continue data collection to document how the changes affect program acceptability, integrity, and impact or outcome.

In the second instance (altering core elements), the teacher's request is problematic given the centrality of student collaboration to the intervention. Using data collected through observation in the classroom (of student group work and teacher facilitation of group work), the program planner and teacher discuss the basis for the concerns. The teacher's primary concerns center on increased noise level in the classroom (which is bothersome to the teacher and has drawn the attention of the principal), the students' difficulty in getting along, and the teacher's reduced sense of classroom control. Several options are discussed with the teacher: (a) address the issue of noise level using classroom management strategies; (b) alter the structure and composition of the groups (e.g., use dyads vs. groups of 5); (c) provide additional training for students in interpersonal process of group work; (d) provide additional training or in-classroom support to the teacher regarding facilitating group work; (e) have someone else teach the class (or videotape the session) and give the teacher the opportunity to do in-depth observation of students' group work (so that the teacher has more direct evidence of what is happening within the groups); and (f) address the issue of noise level through consultation with the principal. One or more of the options are selected, implemented, and monitored through continued data collection.

DA12015; Jean Schensul, principal investigator, Institute for Community Research, Hartford, Connecticut; Bonnie K. Nastasi, co-principal investigator, Institute for Community Research; and David Schonfeld, co-principal investigator, Yale University). The project involves the development, implementation, and evaluation of classroom-based interventions, for sixth and seventh graders, that focus on developing peer norms to support healthy decisions regarding drug use and adolescent sexual relationships.

Adapting programs through data-based decision making in partnership with stakeholders (e.g., teachers responsible for implementation) is consistent with participatory or collaborative consultation. As we have illustrated, adaptation can involve changes in the intervention design (e.g., strategies, content), context (e.g., structural classroom changes; addressing building-level policies), or participants (e.g., staff development). The multiplicity and value of such modifications are supported by research on organizational change and school-based innovations (e.g., McLaughlin, 1976, 1990; Nastasi, Varjas, Schensul, et al., 2000).

Staff Development

The professional development of staff is a critical aspect of the natural adaptation process that characterizes program implementation in PCSIM. Staff competencies are important not only to successful implementation but also to program sustainability and institutionalization. In PCSIM, we adopt a *participatory consultation approach to staff development*, which consists of initial staff training sessions (e.g., in workshop format), follow-up training ("booster") sessions, and ongoing consultation throughout program implementation. Formal training (initial and booster) sessions include lecture, demonstration, practice, and feedback regarding project-specific skills and knowledge. Ongoing consultation sessions, conducted individually or in group format, are focused on monitoring program acceptability and integrity, providing feedback, trouble shooting implementation difficulties, and providing additional staff development as needed. In addition, consultation is conducted in a participatory manner such that staff members are engaged as partners in program decision making as well as their own professional development.

Consultation activities can include observation of implementation, formal and informal interviewing, review of project records (e.g., logs of intervention activities), and face-to-face meetings with staff members. Typically, consultation sessions are more frequent initially (e.g., weekly or bi-weekly) but decrease in frequency (e.g., to monthly, bimonthly, or as needed) as the project progresses and staff become more confident and competent and require less support. The availability of support continues throughout the project but is determined on an individual basis in consultation with staff members.

In enlisting professionals with particular areas of expertise (e.g., specific intervention strategies), program planners may find it necessary to provide them with training in participatory consultation (e.g., in communication, problem solving, assessment of skill level, providing feedback, and training methods). This training would, of course, involve the use of a participatory consultation approach. One strategy that we have found to be effective is the pairing of such professionals with project staff who are skilled in the use of participatory consultation. Working together, these dyads can provide training for front-line staff in the target intervention strategies while using a participatory consultation approach. In addition, the paired professionals can learn from each other. Such efforts also can help to enhance local capacity building.

The participatory consultation approach to staff development is based on our previous and ongoing work conducted in the United States (see Footnote 2) and internationally[3] (see also Nastasi, Varjas, Bernstein, & Jayasena, 2000; Nastasi, Varjas, Schensul, et al., 2000). In addition, participatory consultation includes elements identified as critical to effective staff development, namely, stakeholder participation in joint decision making (Janas, 1998), ongoing support and feedback (Elias, 1997; Harchik, Sherman, Hopkins, Strouse, & Sheldon, 1989; Hilliard, 1997; Kissel, Whitman, & Reid, 1983), and staff empowerment to create change in contrast to the external imposition of change (Murray & Hillkirk, 1996). Furthermore, collaborative models of consultation are effective for promoting intervention acceptability (Kutsick, Gutkin, & Witt, 1991), integrity (Gutkin & Curtis, 1999), and effectiveness or outcomes (Gottfredson et al., 1997).

Stakeholder Involvement, Ownership, and Empowerment

The concept of *intervention–treatment acceptability* in PCSIM goes beyond the consumers' perception of the intervention's utility, feasibility, effectiveness, and consistency with worldviews to include stakeholders' *involvement, ownership, and empowerment*. The goal is to foster full participation and the sense of responsibility and control over the intervention, so that stakeholders come to view the intervention as theirs and to make a commitment to its successful implementation and continuation. Thus, stakeholder involvement, ownership, and empowerment are critical not only to the initial project success but also to capacity building within the organization, system, or community.

The participatory problem-solving and decision-making process described in Phase 3 is critical to achieving and maintaining stakeholder involvement, ownership, and empowerment. The process of stakeholder

---

[3] A 5-year intervention research project, "Male Sexual Health Concerns and Prevention of HIV/STDs in India," funded by the National Institute of Mental Health, National Institutes of Health (Grant No. MH64875; Stephen L. Schensul, principal investigator, University of Connecticut Health Center; Bonnie K. Nastasi, co-principal investigator, Institute for Community Research, Hartford, Connecticut; Ravi Verma, co-principal investigator, Population Council, New Delhi, India; and T. K. Roy and G. Rama Rao, co-principal investigators, International Institute for Population Sciences, Mumbai, India). The project is focused on the development, implementation, and evaluation of a multilevel (community, health care provider, patient) culture-specific intervention to reduce the risk and incidence of HIV/AIDS in Mumbai, India.

involvement begins as initial relationships are formed; continues through formative research, goal identification, and program design; and must be monitored and reinforced during program implementation. Stakeholders can play key roles in decision making about and execution of adaptations, staff development, and evaluation. Through staff development, stakeholders can acquire the knowledge and skills necessary to participate fully in program activities. Development of critical competencies can contribute to stakeholder empowerment and capacity building. Furthermore, the inclusion of stakeholders as key decision makers can foster the sense of ownership.

Essential to the transfer of skills and ownership is the willingness of program planners to relinquish control and ownership of the program. The participatory consultation approach to staff development provides the mechanism not only for developing stakeholder competencies but also for gradual withdrawal of support from planners and assumption of ownership by stakeholders. A key indicator of successful completion of the PCSIM process is stakeholder assumption of responsibility for success or failure of the program and the concomitant perception of planners as superfluous. The process of transferring program ownership is central to capacity building, described in Phase 10.

Underlying the decision making and activities of the natural adaptation phase is the systematic evaluation of program elements and impacts (Phase 9). The approach to evaluation inherent in PCSIM is described in the next section.

PHASE 9: PROGRAM EVALUATION (ESSENTIAL CHANGES AND ELEMENTS)

Exhibit 5.4 includes key considerations for Phase 9. In PCSIM, we adopt broad definitions of program success and evaluation, and use a multisource, multimethod approach to data collection. Program evaluation model and methods are described separately.

Evaluation Model

As suggested by Figures 5.1 and 5.2, *program success is dynamic and multidimensional*. Success is defined by the interaction of acceptability, social validity, integrity, outcomes, sustainability, and institutionalization. In addition, there are *multiple perspectives* on program success, as reflected in the views of different stakeholders. In a sense, success is in the eye of the beholder. Although program planners are likely to have specific intended outcomes in mind, the participatory nature of PCSIM requires consideration of the intended outcomes for partners as well. The inclusion of multiple

EXHIBIT 5.4

Focus (key questions)—Why?

- Was the program successful or effective?
- What is the impact of the program?
- Were program goals met?
- What were unintended positive and negative (iatrogenic) consequences (for individuals, groups, organizations)?
- Were there any unintended negative (iatrogenic) effects?
- What factors influenced program effectiveness?
- Was the program acceptable?
- Was the program implemented with integrity?
- Does the program have ecological–social validity? Was culture specificity achieved?
- To what extent did program acceptability, integrity, and ecological–social validity (culture specificity) influence program effectiveness or success?
- How do the multiple and potentially diverse perspectives of partners (planners, interventionists, researchers; administrative, implementation, and evaluation staff; recipients, their caretakers, and community members) influence program success?
- How do we best use evaluation data for data-based decision making and monitoring to ensure program success?

Participants—Who?

- Program planner or planners (researcher, interventionist, consultant)
- Professionals with expertise in mixed-method program evaluation
- Program implementation staff
- Cultural brokers (who can facilitate access and interpret culture)
- Representatives of stakeholder groups

Tasks or Activities—What?

- Select or develop evaluation instruments or strategies
- Identify and secure existing data
- Data collection
- Data management
- Data analysis
- Data interpretation
- Data dissemination
- Participatory data-based decision making
- Staff development in evaluation methods, including accountability and monitoring

Strategies or Methods—How?

- Data collection methods appropriate to specific program, using multimethod (combination of qualitative and quantitative methods), multisource (from various stakeholders) approach
- Recursive data collection, analysis, interpretation, and dissemination
- Systematic feedback process to facilitate program adaptation and staff development
- Participatory data-based decision making
- Facilitation of participatory process

(continued)

EXHIBIT 5.4   *(Continued)*

Requisite Skills (potential focus for recruitment and training)

- Program evaluation skills relevant to engaging in a participatory process, examining process and outcome variables, use of mixed methods (qualitative and quantitative), and seamless intervention-evaluation process
- Instrument development
- Data collection, management, and analysis
- Data interpretation and dissemination to varied stakeholder groups
- Participatory data-based decision-making skills
- Participatory problem-solving skills—communication, negotiation, consensus building
- Group facilitation skills (e.g., engaging participants in idea generation, ensuring equitable participation, guiding group toward consensus)
- Professional and paraprofessional staff development and consultation skills

Challenges

- Identify or develop culture-specific instruments tied to program goals
- Ensure acceptability of evaluation by stakeholders
- Secure professional staff with expertise in evaluation
- Create seamless assessment-intervention process
- Access existing data within system or organization
- Address ethical and legal issues related to data collection activities
- Secure commitment to ongoing evaluation process
- Secure necessary resources
- Create a sustainable process and structure; build capacity within the system for sustainable program evaluation

Opportunities

- Ensure ecological validity and cultural specificity of mental health programs
- Develop sustainable and institutionalized evaluation system
- Educate stakeholders about value of evaluation
- Build organizational–community capacity for program evaluation
- Engage in systematic evaluation of program acceptability, social validity, integrity, effectiveness, sustainability, and institutionalization
- Contribute to the understanding of how to implement successful programs (how it works; what contributes to its success)—for participating system and larger professional community
- Contribute to knowledge base about intervention effectiveness and deployment of evidence-based programs in real-life settings
- Foster appreciation for the value and necessity of research, evaluation, and data-based decision making

perspectives on other dimensions reflects recognition of the importance of acceptability, integrity, and social validity to immediate and long-term program effectiveness (Nastasi, Varjas, Bernstein, & Jayasena, 2000; Nastasi, Varjas, Schensul, et al., 2000). Furthermore, the emphasis on sustainability and institutionalization as goals of PCSIM necessitates their consideration in defining program success.

The iterative nature of the PCSIM research-intervention process is reflected in the approach to evaluation. Ongoing data collection during

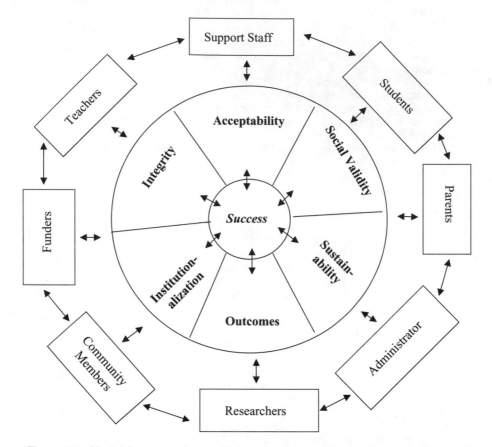

Figure 5.1. Model for assessing multiple perspectives about school-based mental health programs. This model reflects the complexity of program evaluation within the participatory culture-specific intervention model (PCSIM). First, the determination of success (or effectiveness) depends on the perspectives of multiple stakeholders—students, parents, administrators, researchers, community members, funders, teachers, and support staff. Second, the definition of success is multifaceted and reflects the interaction of its components—acceptability, social validity, sustainability, outcomes, institutionalization, and integrity.

program implementation is critical to decision making and activities of natural adaptation and staff development. The goal of data collection is continual monitoring of program acceptability, integrity, social validity, and impact, as the basis for assessing progress toward program goals and making decisions about necessary changes. To achieve a full understanding of program impact, one needs to give attention to unintended outcomes as well. Furthermore, the dynamic and multidimensional nature of program success requires examination of the interrelationships of these dimensions. For exam-

	Student	Teacher	Administrator	Researcher	Support Staff	Parent	Community member	Funder
Acceptability								
Social Validity								
Integrity								
Outcomes								
Sustainability								
Institutionalization								
SUCCESS								

Figure 5.2. Appreciating the complexity of evaluation: School-based example. This grid depicts the complexity of the multifaceted, multisource model of evaluation within the participatory culture-specific intervention model (PCSIM). Theoretically, a comprehensive evaluation of program success involves gathering information relevant to each cell of the grid and determining the contribution of each cell to overall program success. Practically, it requires systematic integration of qualitative and quantitative data. (We are currently exploring approaches to such integration; Hitchcock & Nastasi, 2003; Nastasi & Burkholder, 2001.)

ple, knowledge of the contribution of various program components to outcomes is necessary for facilitating replication and sustainability. Thus, documentation of program implementation (i.e., integrity) permits identification of the core elements of the program (i.e., those that are responsible for outcomes). Similarly, assessment of staff skills in relationship to program integrity and outcomes facilitates decision making about future staff development efforts. Finally, documentation of capacity building requires evaluation beyond the formal program period, to assess continuation of efforts and capacity for program maintenance and future program development.

Critical to both the participatory process and institutionalization are the evaluation skills of stakeholders. It behooves program planners to identify and enlist the involvement of stakeholders with expertise in evaluation. Capacity building is likely to require staff development in evaluation methods, including data collection, analysis, and interpretation.

Establishing a sustainable evaluation process necessitates the identification of existing sources of data, such as key indicators that are collected on an ongoing basis. For example, school attendance records provide data relevant to the impact of truancy prevention programs. Local community police records may include data relevant to community violence prevention programs. In addition, sustainable evaluation procedures may require establishing a system for ongoing data collection within the organization; for example, helping a school district establish a procedure for documenting the outcomes of their social skills curricula or reporting of the outcomes of school-based mental health services.

Evaluation Methods

Inherent in PCSIM is a mixed-method approach to program evaluation that involves the use of both qualitative and quantitative data collection methods. In this section, we briefly describe this approach, with emphasis on the use of qualitative methods to supplement the host of quantitative tools currently available. The focus in this chapter is to provide guidelines for program planners as they make decisions about evaluation methods. It is expected that most readers are fairly well versed in quantitative methods. We refer readers to more comprehensive resources regarding program evaluation (e.g., Fetterman, 1994, 2000; Illback et al., 1999) and research and evaluation of mental health programs in particular (e.g., Bryant, Windle, & West, 1997; Carlson, 1993; Clarke, 1993; Forness & Hoagwood, 1993; Hoagwood, 1993; Kelly, 1995; Nabors, Weist, & Reynolds, 2000; Nixon & Northrup, 1997; Patterson, 1996; Robinson, Ruch-Ross, Watkins-Ferrell, & Lightfoot, 1993; Werthamer-Larsson, 1994). Although a complete description of qualitative research methods is beyond the scope of this book, we have provided an introduction to ethnography as a foundational component of PCSIM in chapter 3 and illustrated the use of qualitative methods for formative research in chapter 4. Later in this section, we illustrate the use of qualitative–ethnographic methods for program evaluation purposes.

Table 5.1 depicts a multidimensional, multimethod, multisource approach to program evaluation that is consistent with best practices for school psychological assessment (e.g., Kratochwill, Sheridan, Carlson, & Lasecki, 1999; Shapiro & Elliott, 1999). The multiple foci reflect the dimensions depicted in Figures 5.1 and 5.2. Similarly, the multiple sources are the key stakeholders who have direct involvement (e.g., recipients, staff) or vested interests and resources (e.g., parents, community members) relevant to the program. Planners and evaluators are encouraged to identify multiple indicators and methods for data collection and to collect data at multiple points in time. In addition to the traditional practice of collecting data prior to and after the intervention, evaluators are encouraged to collect data throughout the course of the intervention and at points beyond program termination to facilitate adaptation and capacity building.

The data collection methods listed in Table 5.1 are consistent with those typically used in school psychology practice when conducting psychological evaluations but extend beyond what is standard practice in experimental and quasi-experimental clinical research. Recommended methods include a combination of observation, interview, self-report or survey, informant (e.g., parent, teacher) report, artifacts (e.g., records, permanent products), log or checklist, standardized measures, and informal communication. Mixed methodology is reflected in the combination of qualitatively and quantitatively oriented instruments. For example, evaluators might use narrative observations in a natural setting, oral responses to hypothetical scenarios, and norm-referenced self- and informant-report measures (e.g., Social Skills Rating System, Gresham & Elliott, 1990) to assess outcomes of a classroom-based social skills intervention. In addition, they collect logs completed by teachers and conduct structured observations in the classroom to assess program integrity; and interview school administrators and mental health support staff to assess commitment to the program and capacity for sustaining the social skills program. Finally, they examine the correlations of student outcome indicators with measures of program elements contained in the integrity measures.

Another example is the use of agency records; semistructured parent and child interviews; behavioral checklists completed by the child, parent, or teacher (e.g., Child Behavior Checklist, Achenbach, 1991; Behavioral Assessment Scale for Children, C. R. Reynolds & Kamphaus, 1992); informal teacher reports; and structured classroom observational schedules to evaluate the impact of a behavioral change program for students diagnosed with emotional disturbance. Data are collected also on variables that potentially contribute to program outcomes, such as treatment acceptability, adherence

TABLE 5.1

Program Evaluation Foci: Definitions, Indicators, Sources, Methods, and Timing

Focus	Definition	Indicator	Source	Method	Timing
Acceptability	▪ Extent to which stakeholders view the program as necessary and appropriate to needs and resources of the system/organization ▪ Commitment and involvement of stakeholders in program efforts ▪ Consistency of planner's conceptual framework with stakeholders' worldviews ▪ Degree to which stakeholders assume ownership for program goals and efforts ▪ Degree to which stakeholders are empowered to effect change consistent with program goals or efforts	▪ Perceptions of program feasibility and value ▪ Type and level of program *involvement* ▪ Sense of *ownership* for program efforts ▪ Sense of *empowerment* to effect change ▪ *Commitment* to program goals and efforts ▪ Consistency with *worldviews*	▪ Participants ▪ Implementation staff ▪ Other key stakeholders	▪ Interview ▪ Observation ▪ Self-report/survey ▪ Informal communication	Pre, During, Post-I, Post-F
Social validity	▪ Extent to which the program's conceptual base, goals, and activities are consistent with cultural values of stakeholder groups and contexts ▪ Culture specificity of program goals and procedures ▪ Extent to which individual outcomes reflect socially valued competences and permit participants to achieve personal goals	▪ *Relevance* to daily life ▪ *Value* in key ecological contexts ▪ *Utility* for achieving personal goals	▪ Recipients ▪ Other key stakeholders ▪ Significant others from key ecological contexts	▪ Interview ▪ Observation ▪ Self-report/survey ▪ Informal communication	Pre, During, Post-I, Post-F
Integrity	▪ The extent to which core (critical) program elements are implemented ▪ Documentation of adaptations (flexible or noncritical elements) necessary for ecological fit	▪ *Critical* elements ▪ *Noncritical* elements	▪ Implementation staff	▪ Observation ▪ Interview ▪ Log or checklist ▪ Self-report ▪ Informal communication	During

Outcomes–impact	• Progress toward intended goals • Accomplishment of program goals and objectives • Unintended impact • Immediate and long-term effects	• *Target* competencies or impact • *Unintended* effects	• Participants • Significant others in key ecological contexts	• Observation • Interview • Self-report/survey • Products or artifacts • Informant reports • Standardized measures	Pre, During, Post-I, Post-F
Sustainability	• Program efforts continue beyond the specified program period • Stakeholders maintain the program when planners leave	• *Continuation* of program efforts	• Key stakeholders	• Observation • Interviews • Self-report/survey • Informal communication • Artifacts	Post-F
Institutionali-zation	• Necessary infrastructure or capacity (policies, procedures, administrative support, staff, expertise, funding, etc.) within the stakeholder organization, system, community to continue program efforts and to orchestrate future change efforts	• *Infrastructure* to support program efforts • Infrastructure for future change efforts	• Key stakeholders	• Observation • Interviews • Self-report/survey • Informal communication • Artifacts	Post-F
Process–outcome links	• Identification of program components (all of the above) that are responsible for program outcomes (as defined above) • Identification of the variables that account for program impact	• *Correlation* between program elements and outcomes	• All of the above	• All of the above	All of the above

Note. *Timing* refers to the point at which data collection occurs. *Pre* = prior to implementation; *During* = throughout the implementation period on specified schedule (e.g., weekly, monthly, on intermittent basis); *Post-I* = immediately following implementation; *Post-F* = follow-up at some specified time after implementation (e.g., 6 months or 1 year later).

to treatment protocol, social validity of target behaviors in school and community settings, and maintenance of behavioral contingencies following program completion. In addition, evaluators examine the capacity for school, family, and community to maintain and plan alternative behavioral contingencies to sustain outcomes and address new problems that arise (see Sustainability and Institutionalization categories, Table 5.1).

To establish a sustainable evaluation process, program planners are encouraged to make use of available indicators (e.g., scores from systemwide or statewide assessments, school or clinic records, juvenile court records) and to develop procedures that can be easily implemented by stakeholders who will remain in the system (e.g., teachers, support staff, parents). This is likely to require consultation with agency administrators about availability and accessibility of data, training of stakeholders in evaluation procedures, and establishing the capacity within the system (or in partnership with other agencies such as universities or research institutes) for data analysis, interpretation, and dissemination.

To ensure valid assessment, program planners or evaluators need to select instruments that accurately measure the target competencies. For example, a global standardized measure of social skills may provide a normative index of student outcomes (i.e., their overall social competence in comparison with same-age peers) but may miss changes in competencies that are specific to program objectives and activities (e.g., social problem solving, social negotiation, or conflict resolution). Evaluation of the latter may require development of assessment tools that more closely match program objectives (e.g., observation of students on playground, response to hypothetical scenarios or role plays) to supplement the global measure. The development of tools does not preclude quantification or the establishment of local norms.

Cultural relevance is another consideration for program evaluators. The question of cultural appropriateness or specificity extends beyond program goals and activities to evaluation indicators and methods. This may require development of specific instruments that make use of the language, experiences, and culturally valued competencies of the target population.

The development and implementation of a comprehensive (multidimensional, multisource, multimethod) evaluation plan is a major endeavor. The capacity of the program staff and organization to collect, analyze, interpret, and disseminate data is a key consideration. It behooves program planners to enlist the expertise of evaluators, to include evaluation as a key component of mental health program development, and to include the necessary resources in program plans and budgets. At the same time, planners need to be realistic about evaluation procedures and attend to feasibility and sustainability beyond formal program activities. Moreover, it is imperative that stakeholders understand the utility and relevance of evaluation data. This requires attention to educating stakeholders about evaluation, demonstrating the utility of data for program planning and monitoring, and disseminating findings in usable form. The inclusion of key stakeholders as partners in evaluation is as critical as their inclusion in other aspects of program development. With their participation, program planners are more likely to achieve acceptable and sustainable evaluation procedures.

Using Ethnographic Methods for Evaluating Mental Health Programs

Ethnographic methods can be used to facilitate culture specificity in program evaluation. In this section, we illustrate the application of ethnographic survey, interviews, observations, journals and logs, curriculum-based materials, artifacts, and social network measures to evaluate program acceptability, social validity, integrity, impact or outcome, process–outcome links, and sustainability and institutionalization. We draw primarily from our work related to school- and community-based mental health promotion and health risk prevention.

Ethnographic Survey

In the Sri Lanka Mental Health (SLMH) Project,[4] we developed ethnographic surveys based on formative data from focused group and in-depth individual interviews (Nastasi, Varjas, Sarkar, & Jayasena, 1998). Culture-specific self-report (for adolescents) and teacher-report instruments were designed to assess the following: (a) culturally defined *competencies and adjustment difficulties* in personal, social, behavioral, academic, and athletic domains; (b) *emotional response* (feelings) to family, academic, and relationship stressors; (c) *coping strategies* for alleviating stress-related emotional discomfort (emotion-focused) or problems (problem-focused or problem solving) and for seeking emotional or instrumental help from others (support); and (d) *behavioral, emotional, or health-related difficulties* resulting from stressful experiences (e.g., alcohol abuse, suicidal attempts, aggression toward peers, or physical symptoms such as headaches or stomachaches).

Students completed written self-report questionnaires about their own experiences. Teachers completed parallel questionnaires to assess the prevalence of competencies and adjustment difficulties in their classrooms and

[4]The Sri Lanka Mental Health Project was funded with grants to Bonnie K. Nastasi, principal investigator, from the Society for the Study of School Psychology, and University at Albany, State University of New York. The project was conducted in the schools of Kandy, Sri Lanka, over a period of several years beginning in 1995. Using the PCSIM, the project team conducted formative research, developed and tested a culture-specific mental health promotion program, and developed culture-specific evaluation instruments. Asoka Jayasena, University of Perideniya, Sri Lanka, was the primary Sri Lankan collaborator. University students from the University at Albany and University of Perideniya assisted in project implementation.

EXHIBIT 5.5
Sample Items for Student and Teacher Ethnographic Survey Instruments

Student Self-Report

Indicate whether each statement is relevant to you *greatly, slightly,* or *not at all* (3-point Likert scale)

- I respect my teachers, parents, elders.
- I help the poor through good works.
- I observe customs and traditions of the country.
- I interact freely with different types of people.
- I persevere even when faced with a difficult task.
- I drink alcohol.
- I persuade others to engage in bad habits.
- I associate with bad peers.
- I criticize others behind their backs.
- I scold or criticize teachers.

Teacher Ratings of Students

Indicate which proportion of the students in your class exhibit the characteristic: 0%; 0% to 25%; 26% to 50%; 51% to 75%; 76% to 100% (5-point Likert scale)

- Follow rules and expectations according to the situation.
- Aspire to a job that will be of some service to the country (e.g., soldier, doctor, teacher, social worker).
- When someone shows them a mistake, they accept it and correct it.
- Move with respectable peers.
- Listen to others' problems.
- Steal.
- Use profane language.
- Are members of gangs.
- Fight with others.
- Carry weapons.

Note. These instruments were developed as part of the Sri Lanka Mental Health Project, with grants to Bonnie K. Nastasi, principal investigator, from the Society for the Study of School Psychology, and University at Albany, State University of New York. Copies of the instruments can be obtained from Bonnie K. Nastasi.

their perceptions of how students would respond to stressful situations. The teacher ratings, therefore, provided global estimates of students' functioning and teacher understanding of student responses to stressful situations. In addition, students and teachers were asked to rate the perceived value of the culturally defined competencies and difficulties from the perspective of students, parents, teachers, and adolescent peer group. Sample items from student and teacher questionnaires are presented in Exhibit 5.5. These measures yield quantitative indices of target constructs.

Our work in Sri Lanka exemplifies the use of existing theory and research, extant research instruments, and formative data to develop culture-specific tools (i.e., ethnographic surveys). The theoretical basis of instrument construction was the conceptual model presented in Figure 3.1 (chap. 3, this volume), the work of Susan Harter on perceived and socially valued competencies (e.g., Harter, 1990; Harter & Marold, 1991), and research related to stress and coping (e.g., Elias & Branden, 1988; Lazarus & Folkman, 1984). In addition, Harter's self-perception scales (e.g., Harter, 1988) served as models for assessment of culturally defined competencies and difficulties. Finally, formative data were used to construct items that reflected the experiences (e.g., academic pressure related to rigorous examination process ["studying for O-Level exams"; students are required to pass O-Level exams to progress to 10th grade], homelessness ["living in the street with your family"], parental drinking, domestic violence, and maternal absence due to employment in the Middle East) and language (e.g., "I *move* [associate] with friends who drink.") of the target group. The instruments were reviewed by adult and student stakeholders, piloted and revised, administered to a large representative sample, and used as pre–post measures in a school-based mental health promotion program. The instruments can also be used to gather information about the general population, to identify needs for mental health programming in specific settings, and to conduct surveillance of these mental health indicators. The procedures used for instrument development and initial validation work in the SLMH project provide a prototype for application to school-based mental health programming with the diverse populations within the United States and globally.[5]

In-Depth Interviews

As we studied implementation of a school-based drug and sexual risk prevention program (see Footnote 2), it became clear that the intervention curriculum content did not necessarily address issues faced by the diverse student population (i.e., urban African American, Puerto Rican, and Caucasian students from lower- to upper-middle-income families). We then conducted individual interviews (Exhibit 5.6) with a sample of program participants to gather data about their social and emotional needs and resources and to explore culture-specific experiences and conceptions relevant to mental health and health risk programming. The data from these interviews, along with data from observations and student workbooks, facilitated modifications of the ongoing curriculum content. Furthermore, these data were relevant to the district's planning of subsequent interventions, thus potentially contributing to sustainability and institutionalization.

Observation

To document implementation of a classroom-based Level I program (see Footnote 2), we used a combination of observation strategies. Narrative

---

[5]Work on these instruments is ongoing. Copies of the instruments and information about instrument validation are available from Bonnie K. Nastasi.

EXHIBIT 5.6
**Examples of Individual Interview and Focus Group Interview Questions
for Middle School Students**

Individual Interview Questions

1. What are situations that cause difficulty or stress for you? [Probe for situations related to drugs and sexual risks.]
   a. Situations that cause difficulty or stress in relationships with peers?
   b. Situations that cause difficulty or stress in relationships with adults?
   c. Situations that create pressure to engage in unsafe behavior?
   d. Situations that create "stressful" feelings of anger? Fear? Sadness? Other stressful feelings [Probe for description–label for those feelings.]?
2. What do you usually do when faced with a difficult or stressful situation? [Probe for personal problem-solving approach and coping strategies.]
3. What "supports" do you have to help you with difficult or stressful situations? Who are the people that you can turn to?
4. What are situations that cause you to feel "happy" or "calm" (i.e., supportive situations)?
5. How do you use "supportive" situations or relationships during times of difficulty or stress?
6. Select specific examples (at least one per category in #1) provided by students and ask the following:
   a. Tell me more about the situation. [Get student's story, describing it in as much detail as possible so that we could recreate a story about a similar situation.]
   b. What could you do in a situation like this to relieve your stress or solve the problem you face? Describe how you would approach the problem. What else could you do? [Probe for alternative strategies.]
   c. [After problem-solving unit in curriculum]: What do you think about the problem-solving steps you learned about in social development class? Have you used them? How are they different from what you usually do? Do they make sense to you? If you could create your own problem-solving steps (e.g., to teach to other middle school students), what would they be?

Focus Group Questions

1. What are situations that cause difficulty or stress for middle school students? [Probe for situations related to interpersonal relationships, drugs, and sexual risks.]
   a. Situations that cause difficulty or stress in relationships with peers?
   b. Situations that cause difficulty or stress in relationships with adults?
   c. Situations that create pressure to engage in unsafe behavior?
   d. Situations that create "stressful" feeling of anger? Fear? Sadness? Other stressful feelings?
2. Select specific examples (at least one per category above) provided by students and ask the following:
   a. Tell me more about the situation. [Describe in as much detail as possible so that we could recreate a story about a similar situation.]
   b. How could you use problem solving in a situation like this? [Describe how you would apply problem solving.]
   c. What else would you do to address such a situation?

(continued)

EXHIBIT 5.6   *(Continued)*

3. What "supports" do middle school students have to help them in difficult or stressful situations? Who are the people that middle school students can turn to?
4. What are situations that cause "happiness" or "calm" for middle school students (i.e., supportive situations)?
5. How can middle school students use "supportive" situations or relationships during times of difficulty or stress?

Note. These interview questions were designed for use in a 4½-year intervention research project, "Building Preventive Group Norms in Urban Middle Schools," funded by the National Institute on Drug Abuse, National Institutes of Health (Grant No. DA12015; Jean Schensul, principal investigator, Institute for Community Research, Hartford, Connecticut; Bonnie K. Nastasi, co-principal investigator, Institute for Community Research; and David Schonfeld, co-principal investigator, Yale University). The project involves the development, implementation, and evaluation of classroom-based interventions, for sixth and seventh graders, that focus on developing peer norms to support healthy decisions regarding drug use and adolescent sexual relationships.

observations, conducted by staff ethnographers, provided in-depth documentation of teachers' implementation of the curriculum (e.g., extent to which teacher follows the scripted instructions and the nature of variations in instructions), student responses (e.g., record of unsolicited oral comments and answers to teacher questions or prompts), student engagement in activities (e.g., extent of practice in target skills, and the accuracy of or improvement in student performance of specific coping strategies), and the nature of teacher support. The school psychologist, who provided consultation and support to the teacher, also completed a checklist each time she visited the classrooms for periodic observation and in-classroom support (e.g., coaching, co-teaching, co-facilitating role-play activities). To parallel the narrative observations, the school psychologist used a checklist that focused on teacher implementation and student response. In addition, the psychologist documented instances of direct support she provided to the teacher or students.

In one community-based substance abuse prevention program for adolescent girls[6] (described in Nastasi & Berg, 1999), we videotaped intervention sessions to provide consultation and follow-up training to intervention staff. Research assistants from a regional university reviewed and coded tapes for use of group facilitation techniques. The project consultant (a faculty member from the regional university) met with the intervention staff to review the tapes and the coded data. The tapes provided the context for follow-up staff training and collaborative problem solving about challenges in group facilitation. (For additional information on the use of audiovisual techniques in ethnography, see Nastasi, 1999.)

---

[6] A 5-year research and demonstration project, "Urban Women Against Substance Abuse," funded by the Center for Substance Abuse Prevention (Grant No. HD1-SPO6758) to the Institute for Community Research, Hartford, Connecticut (Jean J. Schensul, principal investigator; Marlene Berg, co-principal investigator).

Engaging program staff and other stakeholders in observations serves multiple purposes in addition to the most apparent goal of program evaluation. First, systematic observation of key components of an intervention by a participant or facilitator can foster development of evaluative and self-evaluative skills. Second, opportunities for self-evaluation can foster reflective practice. Third, involving stakeholders (e.g., professional staff, community members) in the data collection process can enhance their sense of ownership and empowerment and increase the capacity for program sustainability and institutionalization. On the basis of our own experiences, typical reactions by program staff or participants who engage in systematic observation in naturalistic settings are (a) recognition of the complexity of person–environment interactions, (b) consideration of their actual or potential role in such interactions, and (c) acknowledgment that their views of social interactions are permanently altered.

Journals and Logs

These two methods can be used for multiple evaluation purposes, such as monitoring program acceptability, documenting program implementation and participant exposure to intervention, promoting self-evaluation and reflection by participants, and tracking program impact. To illustrate the application of logs and journals during intervention implementation, we draw from work conducted in two settings (see Footnotes 2 and 4). On the basis of our experiences in these and other projects, we make several recommendations about the use of these methods (see Exhibit 5.7).

The first example (Appendix 5.2) is a *contact log* used by project staff to document daily contacts with students, teachers, and other school staff

EXHIBIT 5.7
Recommendations for Using Logs and Journals as Evaluation Tools

1. Construct logs that can be completed in a few minutes, for example, using a minimal number of items and check list format. Provide additional space for comments.
2. Build time into intervention or consultation sessions for completion of these documents.
3. Collect completed materials on a regular basis, for example, at the end of each session, on a weekly basis, or at the completion of a segment of the program (e.g., curriculum module).
4. Use materials to monitor progress, provide feedback, and identify needs for support or training.
5. Encourage participants (program facilitators and recipients) to use the materials for self-evaluation and reflection in addition to project reporting.
6. Use logs and journals as part of a multimethod, multisource approach to data collection, for example, using other informants and other reporting methods to provide confirming or disconfirming data.

in a school-based project conducted in the United States (see Footnote 2). The log was instituted as a supplement to observation, interview, or field notes to track the type and frequency of contacts on an ongoing basis. The logs were used for multiple purposes: (a) to prepare weekly progress reports to project administrators and school system partners, (b) to monitor implementation issues and identify need for follow-up, and (c) to yield quantitative indices of contacts by frequency and type. The latter indices constitute data about the scope and depth of implementation efforts and expenditure of staff resources. Introduction of contact logs paralleled a change in strategy in which the project staff extended contacts to include building-level administrative and support staff (in addition to teachers and students at classroom level) in an effort to increase systemic support for the program.

The second example is an *activity log* completed by teachers–facilitators in an after-school program conducted in Sri Lanka (see Footnote 4; also see Appendix 5.3). The log was designed to document the completion and successful implementation of session activities, as outlined in the program curriculum, and student–participant attendance. In addition, the facilitators were asked to provide their perspectives on the reasons for completion or noncompletion and success or failure of the activities. The logs thus served multiple purposes: (a) document curriculum implementation (i.e., program integrity), (b) track participant receipt of the intervention (i.e., to compute "dosage" indices), and (c) provide qualitative information from teachers on feasibility of planned activities and need for modifications. To facilitate consistent data collection and feedback, facilitators were asked to complete the logs at the conclusion of each session, and project staff collected and reviewed them on a daily basis. To provide reliability checks of teacher integrity reports and another source of information on the success or failure of activities, project research staff completed parallel forms when they conducted observations. The combined teacher and researcher logs assisted project staff in conducting daily on-site consultation and weekly staff development meetings.

In this same project (see Footnote 4), facilitators were asked to complete semistructured reflection forms at the conclusion of each session (see Appendix 5.4). These forms were designed to encourage facilitator self-evaluation of performance and to gather data about cultural appropriateness and acceptability of program activities. The combined use of facilitator logs and self-reflection (see Appendixes 5.3 and 5.4) not only facilitated consultation and program modification but also provided data about program acceptability, social validity, integrity, and perceived effectiveness.

Curriculum-Based Material and Artifacts

In our own work we make frequent use of the permanent products of interventions as a source of data for both formative and evaluative purposes. Such data can extend, confirm, or disconfirm data from other sources (e.g., surveys or in-depth interviews). The products of interventions can include worksheets completed by participants as part of an activity, written or electronically recorded notes from discussions, self-evaluation or self-reflection materials, and artwork or presentation materials produced by participants. To illustrate, we provide examples of the activities that can yield such products and describe how we used the data.

The first example comes from a community-based sexual risk prevention program for adolescents and young adults, ages 17–27 (Nastasi et al., 1998–1999). The intervention activity depicted in Appendix 5.5 (Nastasi et al., 1996) was designed to elicit problem solving related to avoiding sexual risks. The scenario was constructed from formative research data with the same population and was designed to portray an array of sexual risks. A primary goal of the intervention was the construction of peer norms to support healthy sexual decision making. Improving risk perception related to sexual intimacy was one of the program objectives. Sessions were conducted by peer educators with on-site support from project staff. The activity provided the opportunity for participants to discuss concerns related to sexual intimacy, identify potential risks, consider ways to avoid associated risks, and reach consensus on health-promoting behavioral norms. The activity provided the context not only for promoting consensus building but also for gathering data about participant skill level (group interaction, communication, consensus building, etc.) and progress toward program goals (e.g., creating healthy norms) and objectives (e.g., improving sexual risk perception). This prototypical activity could yield several types of data: (a) individual participant responses, (b) consensual group responses, and (c) the relationship between individual and group responses. Group recorders were diligent in fulfilling their responsibilities, thus yielding usable data. Observations of groups and accompanying individual or group worksheets provided additional data sources to facilitate triangulation. The repetition of similar activities, which provided the context for discussion and consensus building, permitted tracking of participants' progress toward program goals and objectives. Furthermore, by coding open-ended responses to an individually administered pre–post problem-solving scenario, we were able to measure changes in risk perception related to specificity and range of identified risks and link these changes to the content of discussions that occurred during the intervention (see Nastasi et al., 1998–1999, for additional information).

We draw on our experiences in an after-school mental health program for adolescents (see Footnote 4) to illustrate the generation of additional formative data from an intervention activity. The activity was designed to elicit student perceptions of stressors and supports in key ecological contexts (community, school, family, peer group) through the construction of *ecomaps* (visual representations of relationships with significant others; Compton & Galaway, 1989; Nastasi et al., 1999). Students were instructed to identify individuals (groups, organizations, etc.) who were important to them (in the respective ecological context) and depict each person or group in relationship to themselves (the central figure), connecting each with different lines to portray a supportive, stressful, or ambivalent relationship. The ecomaps were then used as the basis for teaching students to identify and label feelings (e.g., associated with stress or support), describe the sources of stress or support (e.g., specific encounters or behaviors), and identify ways to decrease stress and increase support. The ecomaps also provided stimuli for story writing, sharing with peers, and role playing behavioral responses. Not only did the ecomaps prove to be an effective tool for structuring intervention sessions, but they also provided data about stressors, supports, and coping mechanisms. These data thus extended our formative database (Nastasi, Varjas, Sarkar, & Jayasena, 1998). We were able to code the visual and written depictions from ecomap activities using the same coding scheme applied during formative research. Because participants were from the same population as the original study, we could use the intervention data to confirm, disconfirm, and extend findings from the existing data base. Student ecomaps also represent another type of ethnographic method, social network mapping.

Social Networks

The ecomap activity described previously is an example of *ego-centered or personal networks*. In addition to the qualitative coding of content (e.g., types of relationships), the relationship networks can be depicted with the assistance of available software (ANTHROPAC, Borgatti, 1996; UCINET, Borgatti, Everett, & Freeman, 1992). An example of the use of *full relational social networks* in intervention programs comes from an ongoing classroom-based drug and sexual risk prevention program (see Footnote 2; also see Appendix 5.6). Students are asked to complete the pre–post social network measure as part of the curriculum (during first and last sessions). The program relies heavily on the use of cooperative learning as the context for the construction of peer norms to support healthy decision making. The students have multiple opportunities to interact with classmates through small and large group discussions. As the small groups change in composition, students could potentially work with all classmates. To examine changes in student relationships and the social network of the classroom as a result of these experiences, we are using social network analysis.

PHASE 10: CAPACITY BUILDING
(SUSTAINABILITY AND INSTITUTIONALIZATION)

The general goals of this phase are twofold: (a) to foster sustainability of the target change efforts and (b) to enable the organization–system to engage in future change efforts deemed necessary to address mental health crises or appropriate to foster healthy development and mental health of its members. In PCSIM, capacity building is viewed as an outgrowth of participation in Phases 1 through 9. As partners in the development of mental health programs, stakeholders are provided with opportunities to develop necessary skills to assume ownership for the target program and future mental health endeavors. For program planners, this means ensuring those opportunities and gradually relinquishing control of program administration. Critical to this transfer of ownership and capacity is identifying those individuals who will play key roles in continuing current change efforts and instituting future efforts. The cultural brokers identified in earlier phases of the PCSIM process may play important roles during Phase 10.

Principles of Capacity Building

Drawing from the principles and extensive international development and relief work of Oxfam[7] (Eade, 1997; Eade & Williams, 1995), we propose the following guidelines for capacity building in mental health promotion:

1. *Capacity building extends beyond the target program.* Capacity building involves not only sustaining the specific intervention efforts that have been implemented but also ensuring the capacity for continued change efforts. As we have noted throughout the phases of PCSIM, preparing stakeholders to participate effectively in the target program is conducted with long-term goals (for capacity building) in mind. Thus, as planners prepare stakeholders in research, intervention, and evaluation methods, they are also preparing them to engage in PCSIM on their own in the future.

2. *Mental health promotion efforts occur within a social, cultural, and political (i.e., ecological) context.* This ecological context needs to be considered when planning and evaluating specific interventions and long-term programming. The involvement of stakeholders as partners in mental health programming can help to ensure that multiple constituencies (e.g., representing variations in gender, ethnicity, age, socioeconomic status, political views, beliefs, values, and power) are represented.

3. *Capacity building is a long-term endeavor.* The amount of time it takes to build capacity within an organization or system

---

[7]Oxfam is a British nongovernmental, civil society organization involved in humanitarian and development work in over 70 countries throughout the world, with a particular focus on poverty (Eade, 1997).

goes well beyond the school year and typical program or funding cycle (ranging from 1 to 5 years). Building capacity within an organization is easily a 10-year endeavor, thereby requiring sustained commitment, effort, financial, material, and human resources. Unlike well-controlled clinical interventions, building capacity for mental health programs in real-life settings lacks clearly demarcated beginning and ending points. As we have acknowledged, programming begins in the early stages of PCSIM as planners form partnerships and explore common interests, well before formal programs begin. Likewise, efforts continue well beyond the formal end of a specific program.

4. *The road to capacity building is unpredictable*. Mental health programming in school and community contexts presents unique challenges compared with provision of clinic-based services. Similarly, conducting research and evaluation on school- and community-based mental health programs is worlds apart from conducting well-controlled mental health clinical trials. Building sustainable field-based mental health programs with seamless evaluation components requires flexibility, creativity, problem solving, and perseverance. This does not preclude systematic planning and implementation. To be successful, planners must operate with clear goals and a systematic process—plan for operation, but with openness to alternative strategies for achieving goals and willingness to modify specific features and objectives to meet population- and context-specific needs. Using an intervention ↔ research process can provide structure to an otherwise unwieldy and unpredictable process, and ultimately contribute to our knowledge about intervention deployment and capacity building.

5. *Participatory planning and capacity building are risky*. Given the complexity of the participatory process, especially applied to capacity building, outcomes are not guaranteed. Planners have limited control over the myriad factors (personal, social, cultural, political) that impact outcomes and are highly dependent on the capacity and motivations of designated partners and other stakeholders. Unfortunately, empirically validated mental health interventions, based on well-controlled clinical trials, have limited application in real-life settings; and systematic research on field-based mental health programming is scarce.

6. *The ultimate goal and key indicator of success is the impact on the lives of people*. This accounts for the *people-centered* focus espoused by Eade (1997). The goal of school-based mental

health programming is, of course, the improvement of the psychological well-being of students; and we typically measure success by indicators of such improvements (e.g., decreases in anxiety or depression; improved school functioning). Acknowledging the ecological nature of human relationships and capacity building, we extend this focus to the impact on the lives of those individuals who interact with students. Therefore, capacity building requires attention to the impact on the myriad stakeholders who play significant roles in children's lives (e.g., parents, peers, teachers, administrators, community members). Recognizing this, planners assume responsibility for improving not only the lives of children but also the lives of significant others. Furthermore, in conducting change efforts directed toward children, planners need to consider the impact of changes in children's functioning on those with whom they interact and the role that significant others can play in fostering the well-being of children.

7. *Change and capacity building can bring about unintended negative consequences.* As we work toward improving the lives of people, it is important to consider potential unintended negative consequences as well. As noted in Phase 9, it behooves evaluators to document program implementation in a manner that permits identification of unintended consequences. For example, a concern that has been raised about efforts to build peer networks to support healthy decision making in teens is that peer influence could be negative, thus resulting in iatrogenic effects (Dishion & Andrews, 1995; Poulin & Dishion, 1997). At the same time, programs that enlist peer educators have been documented as successful (e.g., M. U. Smith & DiClemente, 2000). Thus, it becomes the responsibility of planners to closely monitor such negative influences and to study the factors that account for positive versus negative influences. Furthermore, planners need to be cognizant of the negative consequences that may result from positive outcomes. For example, teaching children to become more assertive and empowered to take control of their lives may conflict with adult norms within school, family, or community, which encourage children to be obedient and submissive. Similarly, teaching children strategies for nonviolent resolution of conflicts may result in negative consequences when they are faced with defending themselves in violent neighborhoods in which physical defense is valued and necessary. In such instances, planners are strongly advised to consider consequences that go beyond

the immediate program goals and to consider the impact on the various ecological contexts in which the child operates (school, family, peer group, neighborhood, etc.). Involvement of stakeholders in decision making can help planners to address such issues more effectively. Also critical is making participants (e.g., students) aware of the potential positive and negative consequences of alternative behaviors and preparing them to consider such issues when using new skills.

8. *Empowerment of stakeholders, critical to capacity building, is complex.* In the context of capacity building, empowerment involves the development of individual capacity to bring about change for the benefit of self and others (i.e., personal and social change). Just as efforts to improve the mental health of children is best conducted within an ecological context, efforts to foster empowerment of stakeholders requires consideration of the myriad social, cultural, and political factors. The capacity for individuals to bring about change for themselves and others depends on many factors, including personal characteristics, cultural norms, interpersonal relationships, political climate, and power structures (Eade, 1997). Thus, planners need to take a systems-level, or ecological, approach to empowerment of individuals who will be responsible for continued mental health promotion efforts. The process of preparing stakeholders for capacity building is not unlike the process of promoting mental health of children. Both require an ecological focus, with the individual at the center, and preparation of both the ecology and the individual for coping with change. Given the oft-cited resistance to change within any system, empowerment is no easy task and requires perseverance.

9. *The potential contributions of individual stakeholders are not always apparent at first sight.* The hidden talents of stakeholders are not always obvious to planners as they begin the PCSIM process. As noted earlier, the cast of characters is likely to change throughout phases of PCSIM, as different skills and roles become important. In addition, stakeholders, particularly those who are not empowered, may need opportunities to make themselves and their talents known. Planners need to create opportunities, through training and inviting involvement, for a broad range of stakeholders to participate in planning and implementing intervention efforts. Such opportunities for participation can help individuals to identify interests and talents, and planners and those in power within an

organization to recognize potential contributions from a broader range of stakeholders.

10. *Efforts toward empowerment carry risks.* Despite the potential benefits of the empowerment of individuals who are marginalized, there are also risks. Efforts to improve people's lives can be disempowering if success is largely dependent on the efforts of others. That is, empowerment results from one's efforts to bring about change, not by changes orchestrated by others (Eade & Williams, 1995). Planners must take care to involve stakeholders in such a way that they are, and see themselves as, responsible for the changes that occur. The preparation and involvement of stakeholders as partners in change efforts are critical for achieving this goal. Furthermore, empowerment goes beyond feeling in control and capable of effecting change. Efforts to change are not without barriers, and it is important that stakeholders are aware of the barriers and the potential negative consequences of their efforts. To a great extent, empowerment is dependent on the individual's capacity to take risks and address the challenges that arise.

11. *Capacity building goes beyond financial sustainability.* Building sustainable mental health programs in schools certainly requires funding. It is not unusual for grant-funded programs to end when the financial support is withdrawn. Although funding may be necessary, it is not sufficient to sustain long-term mental health programming. As we have noted throughout this chapter, myriad factors account for program success; these factors are important to program continuation. Also critical is a broad base of expertise and commitment among stakeholders at all levels, as well as a systematic process for continued program development, monitoring, and adaptation.

12. *Capacity building is a continual process, not a specific strategy or activity.* Capacity building is not about engaging in specific activities or using particular strategies. It is about participation in a process of fostering growth and development of individuals and the ecosystems in which they live (e.g., families, friendship networks, organizations, peer groups, communities, societies). Capacity building requires continual reflection and evaluation of change efforts by those with vested interests or who are affected by the changes. The notion of establishing a program and expecting it to continue without support or monitoring is short-sighted. Especially when working in schools, the introduction of new programs on an ongo-

ing basis threatens preexisting programs. In addition, staff turnover (e.g., administrative, support, teaching), changing and conflicting priorities (e.g., mental health vs. academic), shortage of personnel (e.g., few or itinerate mental health staff), and day-to-day crises (e.g., episodes of school violence, emotional or academic needs of specific students) often preclude sustained attention to existing mental health programs. Successful continuation of programs requires a system for long-term monitoring and support.

Practical Considerations

Exhibit 5.8 includes the key considerations for Phase 10. In addition to the activities related to capacity building that occur during earlier phases of PCSIM are those that follow formal termination of a specific program. This section is devoted to strategies for planners to use in facilitating sustainability and institutionalization as the formal program concludes.

First, bring stakeholders together to review program data; identify goals for program continuation, modification, and initiation of new efforts; and plan for follow-up efforts. Use participatory problem solving and decision making to facilitate planning of future efforts. Involve stakeholders in identifying and securing necessary resources for continuation of efforts. Ensure that stakeholders from all levels of the organization or system (e.g., administrators, support staff, and direct service providers; students, families, and community members) are involved in these efforts, to secure commitment across stakeholder groups. Encourage stakeholders to institutionalize PCSIM as a process for developing, monitoring, and adapting mental health programs.

Second, make sure appropriate and necessary infrastructure is in place to support future program efforts. Provide follow-up training to stakeholders to ensure their capacity in research, intervention, evaluation, and participatory processes. Identify individuals who can assume leadership in sustaining the PCSIM process. Provide continuing support through consultation for an indefinite period as stakeholders assume responsibility. Simultaneously, prepare new planners and consultants from within the system to assume your role. Help stakeholders identify sources for continued funding, existing mechanisms for ongoing evaluation, and individuals within the system who have expertise related to sustaining current efforts or planning and implementing future programming efforts.

Third, facilitate communication and network development among agencies that can provide necessary resources, for example, between schools and community mental health. Similarly, facilitate partnerships within the school district among teaching, health, and mental health support staff. As necessary, serve as a mediator in building relationships across these and

EXHIBIT 5.8
Key Considerations for Phase 10: Capacity Building
(Sustainability–Institutionalization)

Focus (key questions)—why?

- How do we ensure continued (sustainable) program efforts?
- How do we ensure continued institutional support for the program?
- How do we build capacity among stakeholders for mental health promotion?
- How do we promote ownership by stakeholders?
- How do we promote empowerment of stakeholders?
- How do we ensure the continued use of PCSIM process for systematic mental health promotion?
- Is PCSIM appropriate as a capacity-building model for mental health promotion?

Participants—Who?

- Program planner or planners (researcher, interventionist, consultant)
- Professionals with expertise in capacity building, systems change, organizational consultation, and interagency collaboration
- Cultural brokers (who can facilitate access and interpret culture)
- Representatives of stakeholder groups

Tasks or Activities—What?

- Engage stakeholders in participatory planning
- Conduct stakeholder training relevant to program sustainability
- Secure necessary resources
- Identify or develop appropriate infrastructure
- Establish sustainable process for program development and evaluation

Strategies or Methods—How?

- Participatory culture-specific consultation
- Gradual withdrawal of organizational support, combined with transfer of ownership and control
- Stakeholder training in PCSIM and capacity building
- Stakeholder training in program development and evaluation
- Establish institutional–interagency infrastructure and process for sustainability and capacity building

Requisite Skills (potential focus for recruitment and training)

- Using PCSIM
- Systems change or organizational consultation
- Interagency collaboration
- Expertise in theory, research, and practice relevant to children's mental health
- Program development and evaluation
- Administration and management of mental health programs
- Participatory problem-solving skills—communication, negotiation, consensus building
- Group facilitation skills (e.g., engaging participants in idea generation, ensuring equitable participation, guiding group toward consensus)

Challenges

- Transfer ownership from program planners to stakeholders
- Overcome existing hierarchical structure or orientation of system to establish equitable partnership roles
- Overcome preference for expert approach to program development
- Establish institutional expertise, commitment, and resources necessary to sustain mental health programming

(continued)

EXHIBIT 5.8   *(Continued)*

- Facilitate empowerment of stakeholders to assume responsibility for mental health programming

Opportunities

- Build capacity for mental health programming
- Facilitate systemic–cultural change
- Establish long-term process for systematic mental health promotion efforts
- Facilitate institutionalization of mental health programming efforts

---

other stakeholder groups. For example, program planners in a consulting role can schedule joint meetings between administrators of participating agencies (schools and police department) to negotiate respective roles and responsibilities. Similarly, evaluation specialists can facilitate meetings of mental health staff and school administrators to negotiate a mechanism for sharing information and documenting outcomes for students receiving mental health services.

If the PCSIM process has worked effectively, Phase 10 should be an outgrowth of earlier efforts. To ensure sustained and institutionalized programming, program planners must attend to building capacity as they initially establish relationships, identify goals, conduct formative research, and develop, implement, and evaluate specific mental health interventions. The prospect of institutionalization is poor if capacity-building efforts only commence as the intervention program ends. Related to Phase 10 activities are those devoted to dissemination and deployment in the subsequent translation phase.

PHASE 11: TRANSLATION
(DISSEMINATION AND DEPLOYMENT)

The focus of Phase 11 is the translation of knowledge and intervention efforts to other contexts and populations. Exhibit 5.9 outlines the key considerations of this phase. In a sense, the goal of this phase is to extend capacity to a broader context (i.e., within same community or population; to other communities and populations). The translation process involves three distinct activities—*dissemination, deployment,* and *theory development.* We address these activities separately.

Dissemination

Dissemination involves the communication of findings to the various target audiences, including professional and lay audiences. Successful dissemination requires the interpretation of findings with these varied perspectives

EXHIBIT 5.9
Key Considerations for Phase 11: Translation
(Dissemination–Deployment)

Focus (key questions)—Why?

- What have we learned?
- How do we best communicate the findings, and to whom?
- How can we transfer this process to other settings?
- What are the key elements for ensuring success?
- What are the necessary conditions for deployment?
- What are the implications of the project for theory, research, and practice related to mental health promotion?

Participants—Who?

- Program planner or planners (researcher, interventionist, consultant)
- Professionals with expertise in mental health theory, research, practice, and deployment
- Professionals with expertise in information dissemination and communication
- Cultural brokers (who can facilitate access and interpret culture)
- Representatives of stakeholder groups

Tasks or Activities—What?

- Prepare evaluation findings for dissemination to stakeholders
- Conduct feedback sessions for the purpose of member checking (verifying data interpretation with representatives of target groups)
- Conduct participatory sessions with partners for the purposes of
  (a) disseminating and interpreting evaluation results; (b) identifying implications for subsequent practice, research, and theory development; (c) planning for dissemination to varied audiences; and (d) engaging in reflective activities to consider findings in relationship to personal theories
- Prepare written and oral dissemination materials for professional audiences, community members, media dissemination, policymakers, funders, and others
- Disseminate information to target audiences

Strategies or Methods—How?

- Review and interpret evaluation data
- Engage in member checking to verify interpretation with stakeholders
- Disseminate findings through multiple mechanisms and to multiple audiences
- Discuss findings with relevant professional, community, and legislative audiences
- Engage in reflection regarding personal theories

Requisite Skills (potential focus for recruitment and training)

- Research and evaluation
- Written and oral communication with varied audiences (professional, lay, media, policymakers, etc.)
- Reflective practice or personal reflection
- Facilitating reflective process
- Group facilitation skills (e.g., engaging participants in idea generation, ensuring equitable participation, guiding group toward consensus)
- Expertise in mental health theory, research, practice, and deployment

Challenges

- Secure commitment of stakeholders to the dissemination and reflection process
- Secure staff with relevant expertise (e.g., media dissemination, communicating with policymakers)

(continued)

EXHIBIT 5.9   *(Continued)*

- Communicate findings to multiple audiences
- Secure resources to support dissemination efforts

Opportunities

- Contribute to mental health theory, research, practice, and deployment
- Enhance individual professional practice
- Formalize process of deployment
- Enhance communication skills of stakeholders
- Build capacity in organization or community for mental health programming and deployment of evidence-based interventions
- Establish cadre of local experts who can assist in deployment efforts

in mind. Stakeholders can play a key role in this phase. First, using a participatory process, stakeholders can help to review data, identify target audiences, and make decisions about mechanisms for dissemination. Second, stakeholders can assist in actual dissemination efforts, for example, participating in public and professional presentations, preparing written reports, identifying media outlets, and arranging public exhibits. Stakeholder participation in such efforts may require training and support from planners (e.g., in preparing written reports or oral presentations) and establishing relationships with community agencies (e.g., media agencies) to assist in current and future dissemination efforts.

Professionals involved in mental health programming are likely to have experience in dissemination of findings to professional audiences (e.g., through journal articles and conference presentations). Professional researchers and interventionists may need to solicit assistance from stakeholders to translate "scientific" findings into useful information for other audiences (e.g., parents, students, community members). Phase 11, especially with the assistance of stakeholders, provides excellent opportunities to bridge the gap between research–science and practice. Using creative means for sharing information with direct service providers and consumers, professional researchers and interventionists can make important contributions to evidence-based practice.

Finally, in the spirit of capacity building, it is critical that program planners help to establish a process for dissemination of future mental health programming. Thus, the activities of this phase should focus on identifying and training stakeholders who can take responsibility for future dissemination and establishing links with individuals and agencies to support these efforts.

Deployment

As discussed in chapter 3, a workgroup of the National Advisory Mental Health Council (NIMH, 2001a) has called for greater attention to deployment as an integral part of mental health intervention research. Similarly, researchers, practitioners, and professional organizations have advocated for the use of evidence-based interventions in real-world settings (Kratochwill & Stoiber, 2000; Phillips, 1999; Stoiber & Kratochwill, 2000). Such efforts, however, are limited by the often-cited schism between research and practice. The translation of findings from highly controlled clinical trials to school- or community-based mental health programs requires the study of factors that influence program acceptability, integrity, and effectiveness. Unfortunately, evidence-based application to real-life settings has been hindered by the artificial separation of basic and applied research. PCSIM provides a process by which formative, applied, and evaluative research can be integrated into a seamless process. Consistent with the recommendations of the National Advisory Mental Health Council, we advocate for the integration of basic, applied, and evaluative research through long-term field-based research focused on systematic development, implementation, and evaluation of school- and community-based mental health programs. In-depth documentation of such efforts can provide valuable information about the factors that contribute to effective programming and thereby permit replication and extension of evidence-based programs. A key concept in ethnographic documentation is "rich description" (Lincoln & Guba, 1985), which involves providing an account of program implementation that is thorough enough to facilitate transfer and adaptation to other settings.

Theory Development: Coming Full Circle

As we discussed in Phase 1, a key element in the development of mental health programming is the personal theory of planners, researchers, evaluators, and other stakeholders. During this final phase of the process, stakeholders have an opportunity to revisit their personal theories, consider what they learned during the process of developing and conducting the target intervention, and revise their theories. This, of course, requires opportunities for reflection. Returning to the activities of Phase 1, planners can engage in the reflective process and assist other stakeholders in this process as well. Reflection on these recent experiences and revision of personal theory are likely to influence decisions about future programming efforts, and thus are critical to the capacity-building process of Phase 10. Furthermore, the focus on personal theory, coupled with dissemination of findings, brings stakeholders full circle in the PCSIM process. Lessons learned can inform other mental health research and practice. The delivery of effective mental health services is dependent on the availability of evidenced-based interventions. Using PCSIM, mental health professionals (e.g., school psychologists) can contribute to this knowledge base as they engage in practice.

SUMMARY

This chapter addressed the intervention phases of the PCSIM process. Phases 7 through 11 focus on designing mental health programs based on formative research conducted in earlier phases (Phases 1–6); implementing and adapting programs to meet contextual needs; evaluating critical program elements and essential changes in participants and contexts; and extending program efforts through capacity building and translation. The exhibits and illustrations are provided to assist program planners in program development, implementation and extension activities. In the next chapter, we discuss key challenges posed by the PSCIM process and directions for future research, practice, and professional development.

APPENDIX 5.1

National Association of School Psychologists Survey of Mental Health Programs

Person completing the survey

Name	Address
Professional Title	Phone
Role in the Program	Fax
School/Agency	E-mail

Program Description

Please *attach a brief description* of your program suitable for publication. Do not exceed one double-spaced typed page.

Agency Demographics

Agency Type. Check all that apply.

_____ Public school
_____ Private school
_____ School health clinic
_____ School-linked clinic
_____ Community mental health agency
_____ Other

Location of agency.

_____ urban
_____ suburban
_____ rural

% on free or reduced lunch _____

Program Demographics

Population served. Check all that apply.

____ General population
____ At-risk population
____ Mild adjustment difficulties
____ Moderate to severe mental health problems

Students/clients served:
Total number ____
Gender (% of total): ____ male ____ female
Age range: ____
Grade levels served (range) : ____

Race/ethnicity (% of total):   Clients   Staff
African American
Asian
Caribbean, Jamaican, West Indian
Caucasian
Hispanic
Native American
Other ____

Funding Sources. Check all that apply.

____ External grant
____ Funding agency:
____ Duration of support:
____ School funded

Is program service mandated? ____ yes ____ no
Is program linked to school-based health clinic/
   services? ____ yes ____ no
Is program funded with special education
   funds? ____ yes ____ no
Is program funded as non-special education support
   services? ____ yes ____ no

____ Private agency
____ Medicaid
____ Private insurance/HMO
____ Other

Program Staff

Which of the following are involved in program design, implementation, or evaluation? Check all that apply.

_____ School Psychologist
_____ Certified Social Worker
_____ Certified Counselor
_____ Regular Education Teacher
_____ Special Education Teacher
_____ School Nurse
_____ School Administrator
_____ School Board Members
_____ Other Support Personnel
_____ Other Mental Health Professionals
_____ Staff From Community Agency
_____ Paraprofessionals
_____ Parents
_____ Students/Clients
_____ Community Members
_____ Other

Describe the role of the school psychologist in the program.

In general, what percentage of the school psychologist's time is devoted to the following activities (which may or may not be program related)?

Traditional assessment _____
Counseling _____
Consultation _____
Prevention _____
Research _____
Other _____
(specify: _____)

Total _____ 100%

What percentage of the school psychologist's time is devoted to this program? _____

Of the total time devoted to this program, what % is devoted to each of the following?

_____ Program design
_____ Program implementation
_____ Program evaluation

Describe the methods used by the school psychologist to allocate time for program involvement (e.g., methods to reduce time devoted to traditional assessment)?

Program Goals. Check all that apply.

_____ Enhance social competence
_____ Teach specific social skills
_____ Increase self-esteem
_____ Reduce referrals to special education
_____ Increase participation in regular education
_____ Prevent placement in more restrictive setting
_____ Reduce specific behavioral problems
_____ Prevent exacerbation of mild adjustment difficulties
_____ Increase social problem solving skills
_____ Teach conflict resolution or mediation skills
_____ Increase self-efficacy
_____ Foster appropriate expression of emotions
_____ Crisis intervention
_____ Violence prevention
_____ Dropout prevention
_____ Improve academic functioning
_____ Support school transitions
_____ Parental involvement
_____ Risk reduction
_____ Generalization of program effects
_____ Other

Program Model

Is there a prevailing theoretical–empirical model upon which your program is based?
_____ yes _____ no. **If yes, please respond to the following two questions:**

What theoretical orientations best describe your program? Check all that apply.

_____ behavioral
_____ social learning
_____ humanistic
_____ cognitive or cognitive–behavioral
_____ developmental
_____ ecological
_____ sociological
_____ psychoeducational
_____ psychodynamic
_____ biological/biophysical

What types of empirical information serve as a basis for your program? Check all that apply.

_____ research on program efficacy
_____ research on population needs
_____ research on risk and protective factors

Levels of service provision. Using the following definitions, indicate the levels of service provided by your program. Check all that apply.

_____ **Level I: Prevention.** Directed at the general population and designed to foster development of individual personal–social competencies and creation of supportive social environments.

_____ **Level II: Risk reduction.** Designed to address the needs and problems specific to at-risk populations (for risks due to individual or environmental factors), in order to reduce risk and/or prevent the development of adjustment difficulties.

_____ **Level III: Early intervention.** Designed for individuals with mild adjustment difficulties, to provide intervention for identified adjustment problems and prevent more severe problems.

_____ **Level IV: Treatment.** Designed for individuals with moderate to severe emotional and behavioral disorders, to provide treatment of the identified disorder.

Program Development. Which of the following steps were taken during program development? Check all that apply.

_____ literature research review
_____ needs assessment
_____ adopted existing program or curriculum
_____ modified existing program or curriculum
_____ created a program specific to identified needs
_____ specified procedures for program completion or termination
_____ considered barriers to program implementation
_____ developed plans for addressing barriers to program implementation
_____ considered resources necessary for implementation
_____ developed plans to access or obtain necessary resources
_____ developed plans for evaluation
_____ established criteria for staff selection
_____ established costs in terms of time and resources
_____ established training procedures
_____ piloted the program

Program Implementation.

In what context(s) is the program implemented? Check all that apply.

_____ individual (one-to-one; within the classroom)
_____ individual (one-to-one; outside the classroom)
_____ small group (< 10 members; within the classroom)
_____ small group (< 10 members; outside the classroom)
_____ large group (within the classroom)
_____ large group (outside the classroom)
_____ larger school context (e.g., several classrooms within a grade level)
_____ school context (entire school)
_____ district context (entire school district)
_____ community setting
_____ home setting
_____ other

Which of the following occur as part of program implementation? Check all that apply.

_____ staff training
_____ ongoing consultation with program staff
_____ obtaining participants' (and/or guardians') informed consent
_____ accessing additional resources (e.g., funding, staff)
_____ other

Who serves as referral agents? Check all that apply.

_____ self (participant)
_____ parent
_____ teacher
_____ multidisciplinary team
_____ prereferral intervention team
_____ school psychologist, counselor, social worker
_____ school nurse
_____ school discipline officer
_____ outside agencies (e.g., social services)
_____ other

What assessment procedures are used to determine eligibility? Check all that apply.

_____ direct observation
_____ behavioral checklists
_____ multiple levels of screening
_____ standardized tests
_____ interviews
_____ curriculum-based measures
_____ other

What are the criteria for termination of services? Check all that apply.

_____ participants meet predetermined outcome criteria
_____ participants complete program as specified
_____ participants deemed inappropriate for the program
_____ attrition (%_____)
_____ other
_____ not applicable

What strategies are being used to ensure generalization of program outcomes? Check all that apply.

_____ training occurs in natural context
_____ teach self-monitoring or verbal mediation
_____ reinforcement in other settings
_____ training in multiple settings
_____ parent training
_____ teacher training
_____ implementation by multiple facilitators/educators
_____ booster or follow-up sessions
_____ other
_____ not applicable

Program Evaluation.

Which of the following are components of program evaluation? Check all that apply.

___ acceptability
___ integrity
___ efficacy
___ formative assessment
___ summative assessment
___ generalization or follow-up
___ qualitative data
___ quantitative data

Which of the following techniques are used to collect program evaluation data? Check all that apply.

___ observation
___ interview
___ self-report measures
___ rating scales
___ standardized tests
___ anecdotal records
___ other

Program Outcomes. Indicate (1) the types of outcomes that are evaluated; and (2) program outcomes that have been documented for your program. Check all that apply.

Outcomes	Evaluated?	Documented?
Knowledge		
Attitudes or beliefs		
Target behaviors		
Specific problem behaviors		
Social problem solving skills		
Academic functioning		
Social skills		
Emotional well-being		
Reduction in risky behaviors		
Self-esteem		
Self-efficacy		
Generalization of program effects to other settings		
Maintenance (generalization over time) of program effects		
Move or transfer of student/client to less restrictive setting		
Reduction in school discipline problems		
Reduction in school violence		
Increase in attendance rates		
Increase in graduation rates		
Increase in inclusion or retention in regular education		
Reduction in referrals to special education		
Reduction in special education placements		
Lower rate of hospitalization		
Community outcomes (e.g., reduction in drug use; lower mortality rates)		
Other		

Program Materials. Which of the following are available in written form? Check all that apply.

_____ description of theoretical-empirical model	_____ intake and exit procedures
_____ description of program design	_____ procedures for ensuring generalization
_____ program guide for implementation	_____ goals and objectives
_____ curriculum	_____ theoretical-empirical foundation
_____ intervention techniques	_____ description of program model
_____ evaluation procedures	_____ definition of population served
_____ evaluation results	_____ eligibility criteria
_____ cost-benefit analysis	_____ referral procedures
_____ staff training	

Please enclose copies of program materials.

Additional comments:

Thank you for completing the survey and for your contribution to practitioners and researchers in the fields of school psychology and mental health!

Note: The survey was designed for a follow-up study of school psychologists' involvement in the design, implementation, and evaluation of mental health programs. Results of the study, funded by the National Association of School Psychologists, can be found in *Exemplary Mental Health Programs: School Psychologists as Mental Health Service Providers* (3rd ed.) (pp. 261–265) by B. K. Nastasi, K. Pluymert, K. Varjas, and R. Moore, 2002, Silver Spring, MD: National Association of School Psychologists. Copyright 2002 National Association of School Psychologists. Reprinted with permission.

APPENDIX 5.2

Project Staff Contact Log

Please complete this form for every contact with staff or students, including observations, interviews, consultations, response to inquiries, etc. The purpose of this form is to track the frequency and nature of contacts with school or district personnel or context (classroom, assembly, meeting, etc.). This form does *not* replace observation, interview, or field notes.

Date _____   Your initials _____

Place _____   With whom? _____

Purpose: _____

Questions raised? _____

Decisions made? _____

Next steps: _____

Was concern resolved? (Y/N) _____   Is follow-up needed? (Y/N) _____

Type of contact (☑ all that apply)	Comments
Teacher contacts	
☐ Check in prior to the lesson	
☐ Clarify directions for lesson	
☐ Request for materials	
☐ Information about concepts	
☐ Information about task requirements	
☐ Feedback about student performance/skill	
☐ Feedback about teacher skill	
☐ Feedback about implementation	
☐ Reframe student behavior	
Student contacts (individual or group)	
☐ Answer student questions	
☐ Clarify language (terms)	
☐ Provide translation (bilingual)	
☐ Give examples	
☐ Facilitate conflict resolution	
☐ Facilitate consensus building	
☐ Facilitate shared responsibilities	
☐ Listen to student sharing of experiences	
☐ Give feedback about their work	
☐ Respond to student request for help	
Other contacts (list)	

APPENDIX 5.3

Activity Log

Module #. _____ Session #. _____ Facilitator's name/code: _____

How many students were present today?

[List the students' names/codes on the back of the sheet]

List the *activities* that were planned for today's session:	Did you do the activity as planned? Yes/No	Was the activity successful? Yes/No

Explain your answers:

Other comments:

APPENDIX 5.4

Facilitator Reflection Form

Describe your reactions to today's session. Comment on (a) the extent to which you were pleased with the process and outcome of the session; (b) the extent to which you were pleased with your own performance as a facilitator; and (c) what you would change about today's session.

To what extent was this session *appropriate for the students* in your group based on age, gender, ethnicity, language, etc.?

To what extent was the session *inappropriate for the students* in your group based on age, gender, ethnicity, language, etc.?

To what extent do you think the session was *acceptable to students?* Cite examples.

To what extent was the session *acceptable to you?* Cite examples.

APPENDIX 5.5

Intervention Activity

Instructions to Group Facilitator

- Present copies of the following scenario to group members (in writing and orally). Ask them to identify the sexual risks or concerns the main character is facing, encouraging participants to identify as many risks as possible. The risks/concerns depicted in the scenario include: *loss of virginity; losing the love relationship; negotiating sexual practices (she feels she is being coerced); pregnancy; STDs/ AIDS.* If participants do not identify these, provide necessary prompts to elicit them. Also record any additional risks they name.
- After participants identify the potential risks, choose one risk to discuss with the whole group, using the questions listed below to guide discussion. Record answers on newsprint.
- Then have the participants break into small groups (3–4 members), and have each group discuss a different risk and answer Questions 1–5. Instruct each group to appoint a recorder to write down the individual ideas and group consensual responses to each question.
- Conclude the session with reports from each group and further discussion as time permits.
- To extend the activity, ask participants to discuss each solution from their own (rather than the main character's) perspective regarding: feasibility (competence, control, confidence) and expected personal consequences.

****

Scenario

Female, age 17, B. is the youngest and only daughter in a family of six. Her father and older brothers have jobs. Her mother is working in the Middle East as a housemaid. As a result, she has quit school to take care of the household responsibilities for the family. She has a few friends in the neighborhood she sees frequently. In the last 6 months, she starting seeing a boy (A), age 18, who is from the neighborhood and is the son of good friends of her parents. Because she is alone frequently, A. often stops by to keep her company and has taken on the role of protector. Recently they started having sex. B. is concerned that she might get pregnant because she knows little about reproductive health and birth control. A. says there is no concern about STDs because he is "clean" even though he occasionally has visited a local prostitute. Also, B. feels like she was coerced ("tricked") by her boyfriend into having sex and wants to stop but is afraid he will end the relationship if she refuses to have sex. She is particularly troubled by the situation because her mother is away, she is afraid to discuss the situation with her father or older brothers, and she is concerned about revealing her loss of virginity to other adults in the family or neighborhood. She feels like there is nowhere to turn for help.

Questions to guide discussion of risks:

1. *What is the risk faced by the main character?*
2. *What can she/he do to avoid/prevent the risk?*
3. *How effective are each of these solutions likely to be?*
4. *How feasible is each solution? That is, is he/she likely to be able to carry out the solution? Why or why not?*
   (Using the following questions to prompt discussion of feasibility)
   a. *What skills are necessary to carry out the solution?*
   b. *How competent is the person to carry out the solution?*
   c. *How much control does the person have over the situation?*
   d. *How much confidence do you think he/she has in being able to carry out the solution?*
5. *What is likely to happen if the person uses the solution? That is, what are the likely consequences?*

Note. From *Youth and Sexual Risk in Sri Lanka: Small Group Intervention—Program Manual and Facilitator Guide,* by B. K. Nastasi, J. J. Schensul, P. Ratnayake, and K. Varjas, 1996, pp. 28–29. Copyright 1996 by Centre for Intersectoral Community Health Studies, Peradeniya, Sri Lanka. Reprinted with permission.

PROGRAM (INTERVENTION) PHASES   177

APPENDIX 5.6

Social Network Activity

Instructions to Teacher

- The purpose of this activity is to assess the social relationships within the classroom.
- In the first column, list the names of all the students in your classroom.
- It is advisable to read instructions to students and to guide the students through each question on a step-by-step basis, using the instructions that follow.

Instructions to Students

- The purpose of this activity is to determine how well you know your classmates.
- Please put your name and today's date at the top of page 1.
- You will see in the first column (Classmate's name), a list of all of the students in this classroom. In the rest of the columns are questions. I will read each question, one at a time. Then you are to place a ✓ next to each classmate when it applies.
- Let's start with Question #1. "Who did you know before you started 6th or 7th grade?" Look at each classmate's name, and mark a ✓ if you knew the person before 6th or 7th grade. If you didn't know them, leave it blank. (Demonstrate on the board using "classmate #1, #2, etc.) Be sure to answer for each name on the list. (Make sure the students understand the task. Provide additional instructions and help as needed before going to Question #2. Allow time for students to answer Question #1 for each classmate.)
- Now go to Question #2—"Who would you like to work with on a group activity?" Read the list of names and put a ✓ for those you think you would like to work with. (Make sure students complete the class list before you proceed to Question #3.)
- Question #3—"Who do you hang out with?" Put a ✓ next to their names. (Allow sufficient time for students to answer the question.)
- Question #4—"Who do you talk to when you have a problem?" Put a ✓ next to their names. (Allow sufficient time for students to answer the question.)
- Before you turn in your papers, please check to see if you answered all the questions. Make sure your name is on the first page.

[Sample Form]

Classmate's Name	#1. Who did you know before you started 6th or 7th grade?	#2. Who would you like to work with on a group activity?	#3. Who do you hang out with?	#4. Who do you talk to when you have a problem?

6

THE PARTICIPATORY CULTURE-SPECIFIC INTERVENTION MODEL: CHALLENGES AND FUTURE DIRECTIONS

The application of the traditional biomedical model of intervention development . . . does not necessarily lead to interventions that are adaptable, applicable, or relevant to real-world clinical practices. To ensure that the current evidence base is used appropriately, a new genre of scientific effort is needed to better understand factors that influence the transportability, sustainability, and usability of interventions in real-world conditions.

(NIMH, 2001a, pp. 6–7)

As the preceding quote suggests, the availability of scientific evidence is insufficient for guiding real-world mental health practice. In chapter 1, we identified the critical components of effective comprehensive school-based mental health programs (see Exhibit 1.2). In short, effective programming is characterized by a continuum of mental health services, interdisciplinary and interagency collaboration, and the use of ecological and participatory models of program development, implementation, and evaluation (see Appendix 1.1). Recent attention among researchers and practitioners has focused on the importance of identifying and using evidence-based interventions (Kratochwill & Stoiber, 2002). Certainly, science-based models for service delivery exist. Nevertheless, without models for translating research to practice, the successful application of evidence-based interventions is unlikely. Fortunately, critical gaps in our knowledge (see Exhibit 1.3) are receiving attention from funders and social scientists (Levant, Tolan, & Dodgen, 2002; NIMH, 2000).

In the preceding chapters, we have presented a model for engaging in school-based mental health practice that is intended to facilitate the translation of research to practice and to address current gaps in comprehensive mental health services. In particular, the participatory culture-specific intervention model (PCSIM) provides a process for (a) integrating research and practice in a recursive manner; (b) facilitating adaptation of evidence-based interventions to individual, contextual, and cultural variations; (c) identifying factors that facilitate or inhibit program implementation; (d) developing culture-specific assessment and intervention techniques; (e) engaging professional and nonprofessional stakeholders as partners in programming; and (f) conducting program evaluation that permits identification of active program ingredients. The PCSIM can be applied not only to developing a full continuum of services but also to establishing specific mental health programs (separately or as part of a continuum). The underlying assumptions about participation of stakeholders, interdisciplinary collaboration, research-driven practice, and culture specificity are applicable to the full array of mental health services in schools and communities, and perhaps to the practice of professional psychology in general.

In chapters 4 and 5, we described and illustrated procedures for the implementation of PCSIM. What is perhaps most evident to readers is the daunting nature of comprehensive mental health programming. The process is time and labor intensive and cannot be implemented by mental health professionals working in isolation. Engaging in effective service provision requires garnering the expertise of a range of professionals, integration of services across agencies, and active participation of nonprofessional stakeholders (e.g., students, parents, community members). Building partnerships takes time and depends on effective communication and collaboration strategies. Coordinating the range of activities and efforts of multiple partners necessitates effective leadership and oversight. Comprehensive mental health service delivery is a long-term endeavor. Establishing a comprehensive service model requires careful planning, research, training, staffing, and financial resources. Sustained programming depends on organizational and public commitment, ongoing staff training, continuous monitoring and evaluation, and continued financial support. In sum, comprehensive mental health service delivery should not be initiated without serious consideration to the time and effort involved. Indeed, creating comprehensive services requires the long-term coordinated efforts of multiple partners.

Perhaps most important to the successful application of PCSIM and development of comprehensive school-based mental health services is the commitment of school-based professionals who have primary responsibility for the mental health needs of students. We have geared this book toward psychologists working in schools, based on the assumption that they are in a key position to take leadership in the design, implementation, and evaluation of such programs. Accepting the responsibility for guiding comprehensive programming, however, also requires confronting traditional principles and practices in public education, psychological research, and school psychology. Furthermore, realizing the potential role of school psychology in school-based mental health entails changes in professional identity and professional preparation.

CHALLENGES

The purpose of this section is to identify and discuss potential challenges confronting professionals as they apply PCSIM to developing comprehensive school-based mental health services. In particular, we explore the possible quandaries posed by attempts to institute reforms that challenge traditional notions of public education and engage partners with diverse views and skills in a participatory process. We describe the challenges of integrating research and practice and achieving culture specificity. Finally, we address the requisite transformation of the traditional role and identity of school psychologists.

Negotiating Educational Priorities

Integrating comprehensive mental health programming in schools is likely to raise questions about the purpose and priorities of public education (Nastasi, 2003). Mental health professionals (psychologists) and educators need to grapple with the ongoing challenge of balancing the academic–cognitive and social–emotional needs of students, especially given the current priority of outcomes-based education and academic testing. Mental health professionals need to advocate for the inclusion of schoolwide mental health promotion and health risk reduction programs as they compete for classroom instructional time and staff training opportunities. In addition, psychologists and educators need to work together to effectively integrate mental health and education goals, for example, through creative incorporation of activities that foster social–emotional growth with those that enhance reading or mathematics abilities. Furthermore, mental health professionals have the responsibility of convincing educators and policymakers of the well-documented links among cognitive development, academic achievement, and social–emotional development. Fortunately, psychologists can draw on current educational policies to support the inclusion of mental health and social–emotional development in educational objectives. For example, the No Child Left Behind Act of 2001 (Pub. L. 107-110; U.S. Department of Education, 2002a) and the President's Commission on Excellence in Special Education (U.S. Department of Education, 2002b) call attention to students' social, emotional, and behavioral as well as academic needs.

Engaging Partners

Another challenging yet critical aspect of using PCSIM is engaging the diverse array of individuals who have vested interests in the mental health of children and adolescents. Establishing and maintaining successful partnerships requires ongoing attention to interpersonal dynamics and relationship building as well as task completion. Those assuming leadership for the participatory process have responsibility for fostering open and honest communication, negotiating consensus and resolving conflicts across divergent viewpoints, and ensuring equitable representation in the context of existing power relationships. For example, the psychologist who is responsible for engaging parents on planning teams with teachers, school administrators, and community mental health staff needs to ensure that parents have an equal voice in discussion and negotiation. This may require that the team facilitator monitors group dynamics and discussions so that all team members have equal opportunity to express their views, raise questions, and make decisions. Facilitators may need to give particular attention to fostering empowerment of nonprofessional stakeholders and limiting dominance by professional stakeholders. Finally, working with a diverse group of stakeholders requires openness to different beliefs, values, norms, and language (i.e., vocabulary, meaning). In the next section, we explore issues of cultural diversity that are critical to both engaging partners and developing culturally appropriate services.

Achieving Culture Specificity

As we discussed in earlier chapters, the application of PCSIM warrants reconsideration of traditional notions of multiculturalism in psychology. Within PCSIM, culture is not equivalent to race, ethnic, national, socioeconomic, or geographic categories. Instead, we adopt a broader definition of culture as the unique and shared language, beliefs, values, norms, customs, and practices of individuals. Thus, culture specificity implies attention to the internalized cultural experiences of the individual that are likely to reflect influences across multiple ecological contexts. In addition, culture specificity can be applied to a particular context such as a school, classroom, or mental health team in which the members have both shared and unique cultural experiences. Working effectively across disciplines, organizations, and professional and nonprofessional lines (i.e., as partners in mental health programming) requires consideration of shared and unique cultural experiences. At a minimal level, to communicate effectively, stakeholders need to understand the variety of meanings attached to common language; for example, variations in the definition of "mental health" among parents, teachers, administrators, psychologists, social workers, and students. Moreover, working in partnership and achieving culture-specific programming require "learning the culture" of those who plan, implement, evaluate, and receive services.

Integrating Research and Practice

Essential to psychologists' application of PCSIM is the incorporation of qualitative and quantitative research and evaluation methods with psychological and educational practice. The established practice of data-based decision making in school psychology is consistent with seamless research–practice integration. In addition, the use of observations, interviews, and record review along with standardized norm-referenced testing (e.g., in conducting psychoeducational evaluations, classroom consultations, behavior management programming) is consistent with mixed-method (qualitative–quantitative) approaches to research and evaluation. The use of qualitative (ethnographic) methods, however, can formalize existing practices such as observations and interviews that are often conducted in a less systematic fashion and not subjected to formal data analysis procedures. Furthermore, the introduction of research methods to inform program design and modification can enhance efforts to address program acceptability and integrity. Attention to culture specificity can help to ensure social validity of interventions. Finally, the interactive research ↔ intervention process can contribute to the identification of active program ingredients and foster effective deployment of evidence-based interventions.

Traditional notions of legitimate psychological research and evidence-based practice are at odds with the participatory action research process central to PCSIM. The ensuing debates in psychology, particularly within school psychology, regarding definitions of "evidence" and the applicability of qualitative methods to intervention research (Kratochwill & Stoiber, 2002) reflect the conflicts that those who use PCSIM are likely to encounter. Nevertheless, traditional research designs and practices are insufficient for facilitating successful translation of research to practice and for addressing issues of cultural diversity, and new methodologies are being explored. (For an extended discussion of current debates regarding evidence-based practice in school psychology, see *School Psychology Quarterly*, 2002, Vol. 17, No. 4.)

Changing the Role and Identity of School Psychologists

As we argued in chapter 1 and elsewhere (Nastasi, 2000, 2003), the involvement of school psychologists in comprehensive mental health programming and the application of PCSIM requires reconsideration of traditional role definitions and reallocation of routine functions (e.g., psychoeducational testing). The call for school psychologists to assume a strategic role in school-based mental health service delivery is not new and reflects the unique combination of expertise in psychology and education. Yet, the profession has struggled with redefining the role and functions of the practitioner and convincing school administrators and policymakers of the potential contributions of psychologists to comprehensive mental health service delivery. To function as mental health specialists, school psychologists need to confront current notions of who they are and what they do, and to prepare themselves to assume an expanded role.

FUTURE DIRECTIONS FOR PROFESSIONAL SCHOOL PSYCHOLOGY

In Exhibit 1.4, we outlined the conceptual framework and professional identity of the school psychologist as mental health care provider. Assuming the responsibility for leadership in promoting comprehensive school-based mental health service delivery necessitates adopting an ecological perspective, conducting in-depth study of emic perspectives of clients and other stakeholders, engaging in interdisciplinary study and practice, integrating practice and research in a seamless action research process, and becoming a change agent and mental health advocate. In this section, we discuss the implications of these responsibilities for the future of professional school psychology.

Reconsidering Research in School Psychology

To engage in PCSIM, individual school psychologists need to be proficient in participatory action research and reflective research ↔ practice. This means that the psychologist is continually gathering and analyzing data in a systematic way, sharing data with other stakeholders (professional and nonprofessional), and engaging partners in data-based decision making about mental health programming. This psychologist is a reflective practitioner who continually examines his or her psychological practice in the context of personal perspective, contextual considerations, and data.

The school psychologist as PCSIM researcher works in partnership with professionals from multiple disciplines, including other areas of psychology (e.g., developmental, social, organizational), education, medicine and health fields (e.g., pediatrics, psychiatry, public health, nursing), and other social sciences (e.g., anthropology, sociology, economics, public policy). Effective interdisciplinary research involves not only collaborating with professionals from other disciplines but also using theories and research methods from these disciplines (e.g., theories about culture and ethnographic research methods from anthropology). The interdisciplinary practice of school psychology and application of PCSIM does not necessarily require that individual psychologists have expertise in all these areas. Instead, they must be open to the theories, methodology, and research findings from other disciplines, as well as be willing to learn from colleagues and to negotiate across divergent perspectives and practices.

School Psychologist as Public Mental Health and Public Education Specialist

The psychologist who takes leadership in the development of comprehensive school-based mental health service delivery is one who has expertise in both mental health and education. The school psychologist is likely to be responsible for ensuring that both social–emotional and cognitive–academic needs of students are considered and addressed as programming decisions are made. Adopting the public health perspective endorsed by the U.S. Department of Health and Human Services (1999; see chap. 1, this volume) requires moving away from the traditional role of diagnostician and special education gatekeeper to a broader role that encompasses both public health and public education. The role of psychology in public health has recently received considerable attention (Hoagwood & Johnson, 2003). The assumption of this role warrants serious consideration of the expertise and professional development needs of psychologists working in schools. Moreover, preparing school psychologists to assume the responsibilities of action researcher, public health and public education specialist, mental health care provider, and facilitator of comprehensive service delivery necessitates examining current models of professional preparation.

Preparing Professional School Psychologists as Practicing Scientists in Public Mental Health

Issues related to the preparation of psychologists who can provide comprehensive services to children and families have received the attention of professional organizations, researchers, and faculty of graduate training programs (e.g., Nastasi, 2000; Power, 2000; Power et al., 1995; Power, Manz, & Leff, 2003; Roberts et al., 1998). Questions concerning coursework, practicum, and research experiences have been raised. In this section, we review some of the key considerations for preparing school psychologists in the application of PCSIM to school-based mental health programming. We propose that school psychologists need coursework and applied experiences in the following areas to function effectively as practicing scientists in public mental health. (For more extensive discussion and recommendations for graduate programming, consult the aforementioned references.)

1. Public health, developmental psychopathology, and pediatric psychology, including information about epidemiology, chronic medical conditions, psychiatric disorders, health risks, social morbidities, and the range of individual (e.g., pharmacological, therapeutic), group, and system and communitywide interventions.

2. Organizational and community psychology, with emphasis on organizational and interorganizational consultation, systems change, and capacity building.

3. Ethnographic (qualitative) research, action research, basic and applied research; integrating findings from mixed methodology; and translating research to practice (i.e., deployment).

4. Participatory and mixed-methods approaches to program evaluation.

5. Applying PCSIM to school and community mental health and educational program development.

6. Developing culture-specific assessment and intervention tools.

7. Ecological–development theory (e.g., Bronfenbrenner, 1989) and its application to mental health assessment and intervention.

8. Ethical and legal considerations of interdisciplinary and participatory research in psychology, medicine, and education.

9. Facilitating sustainable large-scale programming through policy change and grant writing.

10. Integrative field experiences in schools and communities that provide opportunities to engage in interdisciplinary practice, research ↔ intervention experiences, and comprehensive mental health program development consistent with the principles of PCSIM.

Providing professional preparation and continuing education experiences in these areas necessitates the collaboration of faculty across disciplines, departments, and colleges. Furthermore, the availability of supervised field experiences requires reconsidering traditional definitions of internship and practicum in school psychology and exploring alternative sites and consortia arrangements. For example, providing integrated research ↔ intervention experiences may require collaboration and joint supervision by staff from university, research, and applied (e.g., school, hospital, clinic, community agency) settings. Preparing school psychologists who can engage in comprehensive school-based mental health service delivery warrants creative solutions from professional organizations, accrediting and credentialing bodies, and university faculty.

FINAL WORDS

At the Future of School Psychology 2002 Invitational Conference, held in Indianapolis (November 2002),[1] school psychology researchers, practitioners, faculty, and organizational leaders came together to consider critical questions regarding the future mission and goals of the profession. What was most promising about this event was the consistency of critical themes across speakers, participants, and workgroups. Using a participatory process, participants discussed and developed action plans to address several key issues that had been identified by the participants through preconference activities. These issues centered on priorities related to academic success and social–emotional functioning of students, parental involvement in schools, and family–school partnerships. Most important to the topic of this book are the overarching themes that emerged. Across action plans (directed toward students, families, and schools), participants consistently called for the following: (a) providing a continuum of services ranging from prevention to treatment, (b) interagency collaboration, (c) data-based problem solving and decision making, (d) continuing professional development for school psychologists and other school staff, (e) integrating practice and research, (f) addressing social–cultural and diversity issues, (g) linking social–emotional (mental health) and cognitive–academic goals, (h) engaging in evidence-based practice, and (i) advocacy and policy change. Moreover, participants stressed the importance of examining current models in professional school psychology practice and training. Underlying the recommendations of participants was the call for systemic reform not only in the culture of schools but also in the culture of school psychology. For example, questions were raised about the need for a paradigm shift in school psychology from a traditional clinical to a public health orientation. Similarly, the question of an expanded or redefined role for school psychologists was raised repeatedly.

Calls for reexamining the identity and role of professional school psychologists have recurred for decades. The critical issue at this juncture

---

[1] The conference was jointly sponsored by the National Association of School Psychologists, Division 16 of the American Psychological Association (School Psychology), Society for the Study of School Psychology, Council of Directors of School Psychology Programs, Trainers of School Psychologists, American Academy of School Psychology, American Board of Psychology, and the International School Psychology Association. Bonnie K. Nastasi participated in the conference as a representative of the Society for the Study of School Psychology. Information about the conference and follow-up activities can be obtained from the Web site, http://www.indiana.edu\~futures

is whether psychologists will be proactive in defining the mission and identity of the profession and take advantage of the opportunity to become leaders in the movement toward comprehensive mental health service provision in schools. This is a decision to be made collectively and individually by school psychologists. We contend that school psychologists are in the best position to assume leadership in participatory efforts to address the mental health and educational needs of a diverse population of students.

REFERENCES

Achenbach, T. M. (1991). *Manual for the Child Behavior Checklist/4–18 and 1991 profile*. Burlington: University of Vermont, Department of Psychiatry.

Adelman, H. S., & Taylor, L. (1998). Mental health in the schools: Moving forward. *School Psychology Review, 27*, 175–190.

Albee, G. W., & Canetto, S. S. (1996). A family-focused model of prevention. In C. A. Heflinger & C. T. Nixon (Eds.), *Children's mental health services: Vol. 2. Families and the mental health system for children and adolescents* (pp. 41–62). Thousand Oaks, CA: Sage.

American Psychiatric Association. (1994). *Diagnostic and statistical manual of mental disorders* (4th ed.). Washington, DC: Author.

American Psychological Association. (1993). Guidelines for providers of psychological services to ethnic, linguistic, and culturally diverse populations. *American Psychologist, 48*, 45–48.

Anderson, G. L. (1989). Critical ethnography in education: Origins, current status, and new directions. *Review of Educational Research, 59*, 249–270.

Anderson, R. N., Kochanek, K. D., & Murphy, S. L. (1997). *Advance report of final mortality statistics, 45* (No. 11, Suppl. 2, DHHS Publication No. PHS 97-1120). Hyattsville, MD: National Center for Health Statistics.

Anglin, T. M., Naylor, K. E., & Kaplan, D. W. (1996). Comprehensive school-based health care: High school students' use of medical, mental health, and substance abuse services. *Pediatrics, 97*, 318–330.

Armbruster, P., & Litchman, J. (1999). Are school based mental health services effective? Evidence from 36 inner city schools. *Community Mental Health Journal, 35*, 493–504.

Arnold, E. M., Smith, T. E., Harrison, D. F., & Springer, D. W. (1999). The effects of an abstinence-based sex education program on middle school students' knowledge and benefits. *Research on Social Work Practice, 9*(1), 10 24.

Astor, R. A., Meyer, H. A., & Behre, W. J. (1999). Unowned places and times: Maps and interviews about violence in high schools. *American Educational Research Journal, 36*, 3–42.

Attkisson, C. C., Dresser, K. L., & Rosenblatt, A. (1995). Service systems for youth with severe emotional disorder: System-of-care research in California. In L. Bickman & D. J. Rog (Eds.), *Children's mental health services: Vol. 1. Research, policy, and evaluation* (pp. 236–280). Thousand Oaks, CA: Sage.

Attkisson, C. C., Rosenblatt, A. B., Dresser, K. L., Baize, H. R., Clausen, J. M., & Lind, S. L. (1997). Effectiveness of the California system of care model for children and youth with severe emotional disorder. In C. T. Nixon & D. A. Northrup (Eds.), *Children's mental health services: Vol. 3. Evaluating mental* health services: How do programs for children "work" in the real world? (pp. 146–208). Thousand Oaks, CA: Sage.

Barkin, S., Kreiter, S., & DuRant, R. H. (2001). Exposure to violence and intentions to engage in moralistic violence during early adolescence. *Journal of Adolescence, 24*, 777–789.

Barkley, R. A., Shelton, T. L., Crosswait, C., Moorehouse, M., Fletcher, K., Barrett, S., et al. (2000). Multi-method psycho-educational intervention for preschool children with disruptive behavior: Preliminary results at post-treatment. *Journal of Clinical Psychology and Psychiatry, 41*, 319–332.

Battistich, V., Schaps, E., Watson, M., & Solomon, D. (1996). Prevention effects of the Child Development Project: Early findings from an ongoing multisite demonstration trial. *Journal of Adolescent Research, 11*(1), 12–35.

Battistich, V., Solomon, D., Watson, M., Solomon, J., & Schaps, E. (1989). Effects of an elementary school program to enhance prosocial behavior on children's cognitive–social problem-solving skills and strategies. *Journal of Applied Developmental Psychology, 10*, 147–169.

Behar, L. B., Bickman, L., Lane, T., Keeton, W. P., Schwartz, M., & Brannock, J. E. (1996). The Fort Bragg Child and Adolescent Demonstration Project. In M. C. Roberts (Ed.), *Model programs in child and family mental health* (pp. 351–372). Mahwah, NJ: Erlbaum.

Bernard, H. R. (1995). *Research methods in anthropology: Qualitative and quantitative approaches*. Thousand Oaks, CA: Sage.

Berton, M. W., & Stabb, S. D. (1996). Exposure to violence and post-traumatic stress disorder in urban adolescents. *Adolescence, 31*, 490–498.

Bickman, L. (1996). A continuum of care: More is not always better. *American Psychologist, 51*, 689–701.

Bickman, L., & Rog, D. J. (Eds.). (1995). *Children's mental health services: Vol. 1. Research, policy, and evaluation*. Thousand Oaks, CA: Sage.

Blakely, C. H., Mayer, J. P., Gottschalk, R. G., Schmitt, N., Davidson, W. S., Roitman, D. B., & Emshoff, J. G. (1987). The fidelity-adaptation debate: Implications for the implementation of public sector social programs. *American Journal of Community Psychology, 15*, 253–268.

Bond, L., Carlin, J. B., Thomas, L., Rubin, K., & Patton, G. (2001). Does bullying cause emotional problems? A prospective study of young teenagers. *British Medical Journal, 323*, 480–484.

Borders, L. D., & Drury, S. M. (1992). Comprehensive school counseling programs: A review for policy makers and practitioners. *Journal of Counseling & Development, 70*, 487–498.

Borgatti, S. P. (1996). *ANTHROPAC 4.0*. Natick, MA: Analytic Technologies.

Borgatti, S. P., Everett, M. G., & Freeman, L. C. (1992). *UCINET IV Version 1.0*. Columbia, SC: Analytic Technologies.

Borgelt, C., & Conoley, J. C. (1999). Psychology in the schools: Systems intervention case examples. In C. R. Reynolds & T. B. Gutkin (Eds.), *Handbook of school psychology* (3rd ed., pp. 1056–1076). New York: Wiley.

Botvin, G. J., Baker, E., Dusenbury, L., Botvin, E. M., & Diaz, T. (1995). Long-term follow-up results of a randomized drug abuse prevention trial in a white middle-class population. *Journal of the American Medical Association, 273,* 1106–1112.

Botvin, G. J., Baker, E., Dusenbury, L., Tortu, S., & Botvin, E. M. (1990). Preventing adolescent drug abuse through a multimodal cognitive–behavioral approach: Results of a 3-year study. *Journal of Consulting and Clinical Psychology, 58,* 437–446.

Botvin, G. J., Schinke, S. P., Epstein, J. A., Diaz, T., & Botvin, E. M. (1995). Effectiveness of culturally focused and generic skills training approaches to alcohol and drug abuse prevention among minority adolescents: Two-year follow-up results. *Psychology of Addictive Behaviors, 9,* 193–194.

Botvin, G. J., Schinke, S., & Orlandi, M. O. (1995). School-based health promotion: Substance abuse and sexual behavior. *Applied and Preventive Psychology, 4,* 167–184.

Brammer, L. M., Shostrom, E. L., & Abrego, P. J. (1989). *Therapeutic psychology: Fundamentals of counseling and psychotherapy* (5th ed.). Englewood Cliffs, NJ: Prentice-Hall.

Braswell, L., August, G. J., Bloomquist, M. L., Realmuto, G. M., Skare, S. S., & Crosby, R. D. (1997). School-based secondary prevention for children with disruptive behavior: Initial outcomes. *Journal of Abnormal Child Psychology, 25,* 197–208.

Bronfenbrenner, U. (1989). Ecological systems theory. In R. Vasta (Ed.), *Annals of child development* (Vol. 6, pp. 187–249). Greenwich, CT: JAI Press.

Bryant, K. J., Windle, M., & West, S. G. (Eds.). (1997). *The science of prevention: Methodological advances from alcohol and substance abuse research.* Washington, DC: American Psychological Association.

Caplan, G. (1964). *Principles of preventive psychiatry.* New York: Basic Books.

Caplan, M., Wiessberg, R. P., Grober, J. S., Sivo, P. J., Grady, K., & Jacoby, C. (1992). Social competence promotion with inner-city and suburban young adolescents: Effects on social adjustment and alcohol use. *Journal of Consulting and Clinical Psychology, 60,* 56–63.

Carlson, C. (1993). The family–school link: Methodological issues in studies of family processes related to children's school competence. *School Psychology Quarterly, 8,* 264–276.

Catalano, R. F., Berglund, M. L., Ryan, J. A. M., Lonczak, H. S., & Hawkins, J. D. (1998, November). *Positive youth development in the United States: Research findings on evaluations of positive youth development programs* (Report to the U.S. Department of Health and Human Services, Office of the Assistant Secretary for Planning and Evaluation and National Institute for Child Health and

Human Development). Seattle, WA: University of Washington, School of Social Work, Social Development Research Group. Retrieved July 2, 2001, from http://aspe.os.dhhs.gov/HSP/PositiveYouthDev99/

Center for Mental Health in Schools. (1997). *Addressing barriers to learning: Closing gaps in school–community policy and practice.* Los Angeles: Author.

Center for Mental Health in Schools. (1998). *Restructuring Boards of Education to enhance schools' effectiveness in addressing barriers to student learning.* Los Angeles: Author.

Centers for Disease Control and Prevention. (1994). *HIV/AIDS Surveillance Report, 5*(4).

Centers for Disease Control and Prevention. (2000a). *HIV/AIDS Surveillance Report, 12*(2), 1–48.

Centers for Disease Control and Prevention. (2000b, June 9). Youth risk behavior surveillance—United States, 1999. *Morbidity and Mortality Weekly Report, 49*(SS05), 1–96.

Centers for Disease Control and Prevention. (2001a). *HIV prevalence trends in selected populations in the United States: Results from national serosurveillance, 1993–1997.* Atlanta, GA: Author.

Centers for Disease Control and Prevention. (2001b, September). *Sexually transmitted disease surveillance, 2000.* Atlanta, GA: Author.

Centers for Disease Control and Prevention. (2002a, March 11). *Young people at risk: HIV/AIDS among America's youth.* Atlanta, GA: U.S. Department of Health and Human Services, Centers for Disease Control and Prevention, Divisions of HIV/AIDS Prevention. Retrieved June 25, 2003, from http://www.cdc.gov/nchstp/od/nchstp.html

Centers for Disease Control and Prevention. (2002b, June 28). Youth risk behavior surveillance—United States, 2001. *Morbidity and Mortality Weekly Report: Surveillance Summaries, 51*(SS04), 1–64.

Cheney, D. (1998). Using action research as a collaborative process to enhance educators' and families' knowledge and skills for youth with emotional and behavioral disorders. *Preventing School Failure, 42,* 88–93.

Cheney, D., & Osher, T. (1997). Collaborate with families. *Journal of Emotional and Behavioral Disorders, 5,* 36–44.

Children's Defense Fund. (1999). *Children and guns: A Children's Defense Fund report on children dying from gunfire in America.* Washington, DC: Author. Retrieved August 29, 2002, from http//www.childrensdefense.org/release 991014.htm

Children's Defense Fund. (2000). *The state of America's children: Yearbook 2000.* Washington, DC: Author.

Children's Defense Fund. (2002, June 4). *Child poverty tops 50% in 14 U.S. counties: CDF ranks worst areas of child poverty nationwide.* Washington, DC: Author. Retrieved August 29, 2002, from http//www.childrensdefense.org/release 020604.php

Christenson, S. L. (1995). Families and schools: What is the role of the school psychologist? *School Psychology Quarterly, 10,* 118–132.

Christenson, S. L., & Buerkle, K. (1999). Families as educational partners for children's school success: Suggestions for school psychologists. In C. R. Reynolds & T. B. Gutkin (Eds.), *Handbook of school psychology* (3rd ed., pp. 709–744). New York: Wiley.

Christenson, S. L., & Conoley, J. C. (1992). (Eds.). *Home–school collaboration: Building a fundamental educational resource.* Silver Spring, MD: National Association of School Psychologists.

Cicchetti, D., & Lynch, M. (1993). Toward an ecological/transactional model of community violence and child maltreatment: Consequences for children's development. *Psychiatry, 56,* 96–118.

Clarke, G. N. (1993). Methodological issues in outcomes studies of school-based interventions for the prevention of adolescent depression. *School Psychology Quarterly, 8,* 255–263.

Clarke, G. N., Hawkins, W., Murphy, M., Sheeber, L. B., Lewinsohn, P. M., & Seeley, J. R. (1995). Targeted prevention on unipolar depressive disorder in an at-risk sample of high school adolescents: A randomized trial of a group cognitive intervention. *Journal of American Academy of Child and Adolescent Psychiatry, 34,* 312–321.

Comer, J. P., Haynes, N. M., Joyner, E. T., & Ben-Avie, M. (Eds.). (1996). *Rallying the whole village: The Comer Process for reforming education.* New York: Teachers College Press.

Compton, B. R., & Galaway, B. (1989). *Social work processes* (4th ed.). Belmont, CA: Wadsworth.

Cowen, E. L., Hightower, A. D., Pedro-Carroll, J. L., Work, W. C., Wyman, P. A., & Haffey, W. G. (1996). *School-based prevention for children at risk: The Primary Mental Health Project.* Washington, DC: American Psychological Association.

Creswell, J. W. (1997). *Qualitative inquiry and research design.* Thousand Oaks, CA: Sage.

Cross, T. P., & Saxe, L. (1997). Many hands make mental health systems of care a reality: Lessons learned from the Mental Health Services Program for Youth. In C. T. Nixon & D. A. Northrup (Eds.), *Children's Mental Health Services: Vol. 3. Evaluating mental health services: How do programs for children "work" in the real world?* (pp. 45–72). Thousand Oaks, CA: Sage.

Curtis, M. J., Hunley, S. A., Walker, K. J., & Baker, A. C. (1999). Demographic characteristics and professional practices in school psychology. *School Psychology Review, 28,* 104–116.

Curtis, M. J., & Stollar, S. A. (1996). Applying principles and practices of organizational change to school reform. *School Psychology Review, 25,* 409–417.

Dadds, M. R., Holland, D. E., Laurens, K. R., Mullins, M., Barrett, P. M., & Spence, S. H. (1999). Early intervention and prevention of anxiety disorders in children: Results at 2-year follow-up. *Journal of Consulting and Clinical Psychology, 67,* 145–150.

de Gaston, J. F., Jensen, L., & Weed, S. (1995). A closer look at adolescent sexual activity. *Journal of Youth and Adolescence, 24,* 465–479.

DeJong, T. (2000). The role of the school psychologist in developing a health-promoting school. *School Psychology International, 21,* 339–357.

Denzin, N. K., & Lincoln, Y. S. (Eds.). (2000). *Handbook of qualitative research* (2nd ed.). Thousand Oaks, CA: Sage.

DiClemente, R. J., Hansen, W. B., & Ponton, L. E. (1996). *Handbook of adolescent health risk behavior.* New York: Plenum.

DiClemente, R. J., Ponton, L. E., & Hansen, W. B. (1996). New directions in adolescent risk prevention and health promotion research and interventions. In R. J. DiClemente, W. B. Hansen, & L. E. Ponton (Eds.), *Handbook of adolescent health risk behavior* (pp. 413–420). New York: Plenum.

Dishion, T. J., & Andrews, D. W. (1995). Preventing escalation in problem behaviors with high-risk young adolescents: Immediate and 1-year outcomes. *Journal of Consulting and Clinical Psychology, 63,* 538–548.

Dodge, K. A. (1993). The future of research on the treatment of conduct disorder. *Developmental Psychopathology, 5,* 311–319.

Doll, B. (1996). Prevalence of psychiatric disorders in children and youth: An agenda for advocacy by school psychology. *School Psychology Quarterly, 11,* 20–47.

Dryfoos, J. G. (1993). Schools as places for health, mental health, and social services. *Teachers College Record, 94,* 540–567.

Dryfoos, J. G. (1994). *Full-service schools: A revolution of health and social services for children, youth, and families.* San Francisco: Jossey-Bass.

Dryfoos, J. G. (1995). Full service schools: Revolution or fad? *Journal of Research on Adolescence, 5,* 147–172.

Dryfoos, J. G. (1998). *Safe passage: Making it through adolescence in a risky society.* New York: Oxford University Press.

DuPaul, G. J., & Eckert, T. L. (1997). The effects of school-based interventions for attention deficit hyperactivity disorder: A meta-analysis. *School Psychology Review, 26,* 5–27.

DuRant, R. H., Cadenhead, C., Pendergrast, R. A., Slavens, G., & Linder, C. W. (1994). Factors associated with the use of violence among urban Black adolescents. *American Journal of Public Health, 84,* 612–617.

Durlak, J. A., & Wells, A. M. (1997). Primary prevention mental health programs for children and adolescents: A meta-analytic review. *American Journal of Community Psychology, 25,* 115–151.

Eade, D. (1997). *Capacity-building: An approach to people-centered development.* Oxford, England: Oxfam.

Eade, D., & Williams, S. (1995). *The Oxfam handbook of development and relief.* Oxford, England: Oxfam.

Eggert, L. L., Thompson, E. A., Herting, J. R., & Nicholas, L. J. (1995). Reducing suicide potential among high-risk youth: Tests of a school-based prevention program. *Suicide and Life-Threatening Behavior, 25,* 276–297.

Elias, M. J. (1997). Reinterpreting dissemination in prevention programs as widespread implementation with effectiveness and fidelity. In R. P. Weissberg, T. P. Gullotta, R. L. Hampton, B. A. Ryan, & G. R. Adams (Eds.), *Healthy Children 2010: Establishing preventive services* (pp. 219–252). Thousand Oaks, CA: Sage.

Elias, M. J., & Branden, L. R. (1988). Primary prevention of behavioral and emotional problems in school-aged populations. *School Psychology Review, 17,* 581–592.

Elliott, S. N., Witt, J. C., & Kratochwill, T. R. (1991). Selecting, implementing, and evaluating classroom interventions. In G. Stoner, M. R. Shinn, & H. M. Walker (Eds.), *Interventions for achievement and behavior problems* (pp. 99–135). Silver Spring, MD: National Association of School Psychologists.

Evans, S. W. (1999). Mental health services in schools: Utilization, effectiveness, and consent. *Clinical Psychology Review, 19,* 165–178.

Farrell, A. D., & Meyer, A. L. (1997). The effectiveness of a school-based curriculum for reducing violence among urban sixth-grade students. *American Journal of Public Health, 87,* 979–984.

Federal Interagency Forum on Child and Family Statistics. (1997). *America's children: Key national indicators of well-being, 1997.* Washington, DC: U.S. Government Printing Office.

Federal Interagency Forum on Child and Family Statistics. (2001). *America's children: Key national indicators of well-being, 2001.* Washington, DC: U.S. Government Printing Office.

Fetterman, D. M. (1994). Steps of empowerment evaluation: From California to Cape Town. *Education and Program Planning, 17,* 305–313.

Fetterman, D. M. (2000). *Foundations of empowerment evaluation.* Thousand Oaks, CA: Sage.

Flaherty, L. T., & Weist, M. D. (1999). School-based mental health services: The Baltimore models. *Psychology in the Schools, 36,* 379–389.

Fletcher, K. E. (1996). Childhood posttraumatic disorder. In E. J. Marsh & R. A. Barkley (Eds.), *Child psychopathology* (pp. 242–276). New York: Guilford Press.

Forness, S. R., & Hoagwood, K. (1993). Where angels fear to tread: Issues in sampling, design, and implementation of school-based mental health services research. *School Psychology Quarterly, 8,* 291–300.

Friedman, M. J., & Marsella, A. J. (1996). Posttraumatic stress disorder: An overview of the concept. In A. J. Marsella, M. J. Friedman, E. T. Gerrity, & R. M. Scurfield (Eds.), *Ethnocultural aspects of posttraumatic stress disorder: Issues, research, and clinical applications* (pp. 11–32). Washington, DC: American Psychological Association.

Friend, M., & Cook, L. (1996). *Interactions: Collaboration skills for school professionals* (2nd ed.). White Plains, NY: Longman.

Garrison, E. G., Roy, I. S., & Azar, V. (1999). Responding to mental health needs of Latino children and families through school-based services. *Clinical Psychology Review, 19,* 199–219.

Gayle, H., Manoff, S., & Rogers, M. (1989, June). *Epidemiology of AIDS in adolescents, USA*. Paper presented at the Fifth International AIDS Conference, Montreal, Quebec, Canada.

Gottfredson, D. C., Fink, C. M., Skroban, S., & Gottfredson, G. D. (1997). Making prevention work. In R. P. Weissberg, T. P. Gullotta, R. L. Hampton, B. A. Ryan, & G. R. Adams (Eds.), *Healthy Children 2010: Establishing preventive services* (pp. 219–252). Thousand Oaks, CA: Sage.

Graham, D. S. (1998). Consultation effectiveness and treatment acceptability: An examination of consultee requests and consultant responses. *School Psychology Quarterly, 13*, 155–168.

Greenberg, M. T., Domitrovich, C., & Bumbarger, B. (2000, June). *Preventing mental disorders in school-age children: A review of effectiveness of prevention programs* (Report to U.S. Department of Health and Human Services, Substance Abuse Mental Health Services Administration, Center for Mental Health Services). University Park: Pennsylvania State University, College of Health and Human Development, Prevention Research Center for the Promotion of Human Development.

Greenwood, D. J., Whyte, W. F., & Harkavy, I. (1993). Participatory action research as a process and as a goal. *Human Relations, 46*, 175–192.

Gresham, F. M. (1998). Social skills training: Should we raze, remodel, or rebuild? *Behavioral Disorders, 24*, 19–25.

Gresham, F. M., & Elliott, S. N. (1990). *Social Skills Rating System manual*. Circle Pines, MN: American Guidance Service.

Guisinger, S., & Blatt, S. J. (1994). Individuality and relatedness: Evolution of a fundamental dialectic. *American Psychologist, 49*, 104–111.

Gutkin, T. B., & Curtis, M. J. (1999). School-based consultation theory and practice: The art and science of indirect service delivery. In C. R. Reynolds & T. B. Gutkin (Eds.), *Handbook of school psychology* (3rd ed., pp. 598–637). New York: Wiley.

Hannah, F. P., & Nichol, G. T. (1996). Memphis city schools mental health center. In M. C. Roberts (Ed.), *Model programs in child and family mental health* (pp. 173–192). Mahwah, NJ: Erlbaum.

Harchik, A. E., Sherman, J. A., Hopkins, B. L., Strouse, M. C., & Sheldon, J. B. (1989). Use of behavioral techniques by paraprofessional staff: A review and proposal. *Behavioral Residential Treatment, 4*, 331–357.

Harold, R. D., & Harold, N. B. (1993). School-based clinics: A response to the physical and mental health needs of adolescents. *Health and Social Work, 18*, 65–74.

Harter, S. (1988). *Manual for the Self-Perception Profile for Adolescents*. Denver, CO: University of Denver.

Harter, S. (1990). Processes underlying adolescent self-concept formation. In R. Montemayor, G. R. Adams, & T. P. Gullotta (Eds.), *From childhood to adolescence: A transitional period?* (pp. 205–239). Newbury Park, CA: Sage.

Harter, S. (1999). *The construction of the self: A developmental perspective*. New York: Guilford Press.

Harter, S., & Marold, D. B. (1991). A model of determinants and mediational role of self-worth: Implications for adolescent depression and suicidal ideation. In J. Strauss & G. R. Goethals (Eds.), *The self: Interdisciplinary approaches* (pp. 66–92). New York: Springer-Verlag.

Hawkins, J. D., Catalano, R. F., & Miller, J. Y. (1992). Risk and protective factors for alcohol and other drug problems in adolescence and early adulthood: Implications for substance abuse prevention. *Psychological Bulletin, 112*, 64–105.

Haynes, N. M., & Comer, J. P. (1996). Integrating schools, families, and communities through successful school reform: The School Development Project. *School Psychology Review, 25*, 501–506.

Heflinger, C. A., & Bickman, L. (1996). Family empowerment: A conceptual model for promoting parent–professional partnership. In C. A. Heflinger & C. T. Nixon (Eds.), *Children's mental health services: Vol. 2: Families and the mental health system for children and adolescents* (pp. 96–116). Thousand Oaks, CA: Sage.

Hermans, H. J. M., & Kempen, H. J. G. (1998). Moving cultures: The perilous problems of cultural dichotomies in a globalizing society. *American Psychologist, 53*, 1111–1120.

Hilliard, A., III. (1997). The structure of valid staff development. *Journal of Staff Development, 18*, 28–34.

Hitchock, J., & Nastasi, B. K. (2003, April). Identifying and validating culturally specific emic factors relevant to self-concept: Methodological considerations. In B. Nastasi (Chair), *Social–emotional learning in schools: Conceptual, methodological, policy, and practice issues*. Symposium conducted at the annual meeting of the American Educational Research Association, Chicago.

Hoagwood, K. (1993). Introduction: Methodological issues in school-based mental health services research. *School Psychology Quarterly, 8*, 239–240.

Hoagwood, K., & Erwin, H. D. (1997). Effectiveness of school-based mental health services for children: A 10-year research review. *Journal of Child and Family Studies, 6*, 435–451.

Hoagwood, K., Jensen, P. S., Petti, T., & Burns, B. J. (1996). Outcomes of mental health care for children and adolescents: I. A comprehensive conceptual model. *Journal of American Academy of Child and Adolescent Psychiatry, 35*, 1055–1063.

Hoagwood, K., & Johnson, J. (2003). School psychology: A public health framework: I. From evidence-based practices to evidence-based policies. *Journal of School Psychology, 41*, 3–22.

Holtzman, W. H. (1997). Community psychology and full-service schools in different cultures. *American Psychologist, 52*, 381–389.

Hoshmand, L. T., & Polkinghorne, D. E. (1992). Redefining the science–practice relationship and professional training. *American Psychologist, 47*, 55–66.

Howard, K. A., Flora, J., & Griffin, M. (1999). Violence-prevention programs in schools: State of the science and implications for future research. *Applied and Preventive Psychology, 8,* 197–215.

Illback, R. J., Zins, J. E., & Maher, C. A. (1999). Program planning and evaluation: Principles, procedures, and planned change. In C. R. Reynolds & T. B. Gutkin (Eds.), *Handbook of school psychology* (3rd ed., pp. 907–932). New York: Wiley.

Ingraham, C. L. (2000). Consultation through a multicultural lens: Multicultural and cross-cultural consultation in schools. *School Psychology Review, 29,* 320–343.

Janas, M. (1998). Shhhh, the dragon is asleep and its name is resistance. *Journal of Staff Development, 19,* 13–16.

Jennings, J., Pearson, G., & Harris, M. (2000). Implementing and maintaining school-based mental health services in a large, urban school district. *Journal of School Health, 70,* 201–205.

Johnston, L. D., O'Malley, P. M., & Bachman, J. G. (2001a). *The Monitoring the Future national survey results on adolescent drug use: Overview of key findings, 2000* (NIH Publication No. 01-4923). Bethesda, MD: National Institute on Drug Abuse.

Johnston, L. D., O'Malley, P. M., & Bachman, J. G. (2001b). *The Monitoring the Future national survey results on drug use, 1975–2000: Vol. I. Secondary school students* (NIH Publication No. 01-4924). Bethesda, MD: National Institute on Drug Abuse.

Jordan, D. (1996). The Ventura Planning Model: Lessons in reforming a system. In M. C. Roberts (Ed.), *Model programs in child and family mental health* (pp. 373–390). Mahwah, NJ: Erlbaum.

Kaltiala-Heino, R., Rimpela, M., Rantanen, P., & Rimpela, A. (2000). Bullying at school: An indicator of adolescents at risk for mental disorders. *Journal of Adolescence, 23,* 661–674.

Kamps, D. M., & Tankersley, M. (1996). Prevention of behavioral and conduct disorders: Trends and research issues. *Behavioral Disorders, 22,* 41–48.

Kann, L., Anderson, J. E., Holtzman, D., Ross, J., Truman, B. I., Collins, J., & Kolbe, L. J. (1991). HIV-related knowledge, beliefs, and behaviors among high school students in the United States: Results from a national survey. *Journal of School Health, 61,* 397–401.

Kay, P. J., & Fitzgerald, M. F. (1997). Parents + teachers + action research = real involvement. *Teaching Exceptional Children, 30,* 8–11.

Kazdin, A. E., Bass, D., Ayers, W. A., & Rodgers, A. (1990). Empirical and clinical focus of child and adolescent psychotherapy research. *Journal of Consulting and Clinical Psychology, 58,* 729–740.

Kelly, J. A. (1995). *Changing HIV risk behavior: Practical strategies.* New York: Guilford Press.

Kemmis, S., & McTaggart, R. (2000). Participatory action research. In N. K. Denzin & Y. S. Lincoln (Eds.), *Handbook of qualitative research* (2nd ed., pp. 567–605). Thousand Oaks, CA: Sage.

Kirby, D., Resnick, M. D., Downes, B., Kocher, T., Gunderson, P., Potthoff, S., et al. (1993). The effects of school-based health clinics in St. Paul on school-wide birthrates. *Family Planning Perspectives, 25,* 12–16.

Kissel, R. C., Whitman, T. L., & Reid, D. H. (1983). An institutional staff training and self-management program for developing multiple self-care skills in severely/profoundly retarded individuals. *Journal of Applied Behavior Analysis, 16,* 395–415.

Klein, J. D., & Cox, E. M. (1995). School-based health clinics in the mid-1990s. *Current Opinion in Pediatrics, 7,* 353–359.

Klingman, A. (1996). School-based intervention in disaster and trauma. In M. C. Roberts (Ed.), *Model programs in child and family mental health* (pp. 149–173). Mahwah, NJ: Erlbaum.

Knoff, H. M. (1996). The interface of school, community, and health care reform: Organizational directions toward effective services for children and youth. *School Psychology Review, 25,* 446–464.

Knoff, H. M., & Batsche, G. M. (1995). Project ACHIEVE: Analyzing a school reform process for at-risk and underachieving students. *School Psychology Review, 24,* 579–603.

Kochanek, M. A., Smith, B. L., & Anderson, R. N. (1999). Deaths: Preliminary data for 1999. *National Vital Statistics Report, 49*(3).

Kolbe, L. J., Collins, J., & Cortese, P. (1997). Building the capacity of schools to improve the health of the nation: A call for assistance from psychologists. *American Psychologist, 52,* 256–265.

Kotkin, R. (1998). The Irvine Paraprofessional Program: Promising practice for serving students with ADHD. *Journal of Learning Disabilities, 31,* 556–565.

Kratochwill, T. R., Sheridan, S. M., Carlson, J., & Lasecki, K. L. (1999). Advances in behavioral assessment. In C. R. Reynolds & T. B. Gutkin (Eds.), *Handbook of school psychology* (3rd ed., pp. 350–382). New York: Wiley.

Kratochwill, T. R., & Stoiber, K. C. (2000). Empirically supported interventions and school psychology: Conceptual and practice issues—Part II. *School Psychology Quarterly, 15,* 233–253.

Kratochwill, T. R., & Stoiber, K. C. (2002). Evidence-based interventions in school psychology: Conceptual foundations of the *Procedural and Coding Manual* of Division 16 and the Society for the Study of School Psychology Task Force. *School Psychology Quarterly, 17,* 341–389.

Kubiszyn, T. (1999). Integrating health and mental health services in schools: Psychologists collaborating with primary care providers. *Clinical Psychology Review, 19,* 179–198.

Kutsick, K. A., Gutkin, T. B., & Witt, J. C. (1991). The impact of treatment development process, intervention type, and problem severity on treatment acceptability as judged by classroom teachers. *Psychology in the Schools, 28,* 325–331.

Landua, S., Pryor, J. B., & Haefli, K. (1995). Pediatric HIV: School-based sequelae and curricular interventions for infection prevention and social acceptance. *School Psychology Review, 24,* 213–229.

Laurent, J., Hadler, J. R., & Stark, K. D. (1994). A multiple-stage screening procedure for the identification of childhood anxiety disorders. *School Psychology Quarterly, 9,* 239–255.

Lazarus, R. S., & Folkman, S. (1984). *Stress, appraisal, and coping.* New York: Springer.

LeCompte, M. D., & Schensul, S. S. (1999). *Analyzing and interpreting ethnographic data: Ethnographer's toolkit, Book 5.* Walnut Creek, CA: AltaMira.

Leff, S. S. (2001, August). Establishing community partnerships to prevent aggression: The PLAYS Program. In T. J. Power (Chair), *Building community partnerships to link research into practice in urban schools.* Symposium conducted at the 109th Annual Convention of the American Psychological Association, San Francisco.

Levant, R. F., Tolan, P., & Dodgen, D. (2002). New directions in children's mental health policy: Psychology's role. *Professional Psychology: Research and Practice, 33,* 115–124.

Leviton, L. C. (1996). Integrating psychology and public health: Challenges and opportunities. *American Psychologist, 51,* 42–51.

Lincoln, Y. S., & Guba, E. G. (1985). *Naturalistic inquiry.* Thousand Oaks, CA: Sage.

Lonigan, C. J., Elbert, J. C., & Johnson, S. B. (1998). Empirically supported psychosocial interventions for children: An overview. *Journal of Clinical Child Psychology, 27,* 138–145.

Malley, P. B., Kush, F., & Bogo, G. M. (1994). School-based adolescent suicide prevention and intervention programs: A survey. *The School Counselor, 42,* 130–136.

Mazza, J. J. (1997). School-based suicide prevention programs: Are They Effective? *School Psychology Review, 26,* 382–396.

Mazza, J. J., & Overstreet, S. (2000). Children and adolescents exposed to community violence: A mental health perspective for school psychologists. *School Psychology Review, 29,* 86–101.

Mazza, J. J., & Reynolds, W. M. (1999). Exposure to violence in inner-city adolescents: Relationships of suicidal ideation, depression, and PTSD symptomatology. *Journal of Abnormal Child Psychology, 27,* 203–214.

McConaughy, S. H., Kay, P. J., & Fitzgerald, M. (1999). The achieving, behaving, caring project for preventing ED: Two-year outcomes. *Journal of Emotional and Behavioral Disorders, 7,* 224–239.

McCord, M. T., Klein, J. D., Foy, J. M., & Fothergill, K. (1993). School-based clinic use and school performance. *Journal of Adolescent Health, 14,* 91–98.

McDonald, L., & Sayger, T. V. (1998). Impact of a family and school based prevention program on protective factors for high risk youth. *Drugs and Society, 12*(1/2), 61–85.

McLaughlin, M. W. (1976). Implementation as mutual adaptation: Change in classroom organization. *Teachers College Record, 77*, 340–351.

McLaughlin, M. W. (1990). The Rand Change Agent Study revisited: Macro perspectives and micro realities. *Educational Researcher, 19*(9), 11–16.

Meyers, J., & Nastasi, B. K. (1998). Primary prevention in school settings. In C. R. Reynolds & T. B. Gutkin (Eds.), *Handbook of school psychology* (3rd ed., pp. 764–799). New York: Wiley.

Miles, M. B., & Huberman, A. M. (1994). *Qualitative data analysis* (2nd ed.). Thousand Oaks, CA: Sage.

Miller, G. E., Brehm, K., & Whitehouse, S. (1998). Reconceptualizing school-based prevention for antisocial behavior within a resiliency framework. *School Psychology Review, 27*, 364–379.

Moore, K. A., Sugland, B. W., Blumenthal, C., Glei, D., & Snyder, N. (1995). *Adolescent pregnancy prevention programs: Interventions and evaluations*. Washington, DC: Child Trends.

Mortenson, B. P., & Witt, J. C. (1998). The use of weekly performance feedback to increase teacher implementation of a prereferral academic intervention. *School Psychology Review, 27*, 613–627.

Murray, S., & Hillkirk, K. (1996). Moving a small rural high school toward self-renewal. *Journal of Staff Development, 17*, 46–50.

Mynard, H., Joseph, S., & Alexander, J. (2000). Peer-victimization and posttraumatic stress in adolescents. *Personality and Individual Differences, 29*, 815–821.

Nabors, L. A., Reynolds, M. W., & Weist, M. D. (2000). Qualitative evaluation of high school mental health program. *Journal of Youth and Adolescence, 29*(1), 1–13.

Nabors, L. A., Weist, M. D., Holden, E. W., & Tashman, N. A. (1999). Quality service provision in children's mental health care. *Children's Services: Social Policy Research, and Practice, 2*(2), 57–79.

Nabors, L. A., Weist, M. D., & Reynolds, M. W. (2000). Overcoming challenges in outcome evaluations of school mental health programs. *Journal of School Health, 70*, 206–209.

Nastasi, B. K. (1995). Is early identification of children of alcoholics necessary for preventive intervention? Reaction to Havey & Dodd. *Journal of School Psychology, 33*, 327–335.

Nastasi, B. K. (1998). A model for mental health programming in schools and communities. *School Psychology Review, 27*, 165–174.

Nastasi, B. K. (1999). Audiovisual methods in ethnography. In J. J. Schensul & M. D. LeCompte (Eds.), *Enhanced ethnographic techniques: Audiovisual techniques, focused group interviews, and elicitation techniques—Ethnographer's toolkit, Book 3* (pp. 1–50). Walnut Creek, CA: AltaMira.

Nastasi, B. K. (2000). School psychologists as health-care providers in the 21st century: Conceptual framework, professional identity, and professional practice. *School Psychology Review, 29*, 540–554.

Nastasi, B. K. (2003). Commentary: Challenges in forging partnerships to advance mental health science and practice. *School Psychology Review, 32*, 48–52.

Nastasi, B. K. (2004). Mental health promotion. In R. Brown (Ed.), *Handbook of pediatric psychology in school settings*. Mahwah, NJ: Erlbaum.

Nastasi, B. K., & Berg, M. (1999). Using ethnography to strengthen and evaluate intervention programs. In J. J. Schensul & M. D. LeCompte (Eds.), *The ethnographer's toolkit—Book 7: Using ethnographic data: Interventions, public programming, and public policy* (pp. 1–56). Walnut Creek, CA: AltaMira Press.

Nastasi, B. K., & Burkholder, G. (2001, August). The child's perspective on interventions: Methodological considerations. In B. Nastasi (Chair), *Do researchers care what children and adolescents think about interventions?* Symposium conducted at the 109th Annual Convention of the American Psychological Association, San Francisco.

Nastasi, B. K., & DeZolt, D. M. (1994). *School interventions for children of alcoholics*. New York: Guilford Press.

Nastasi, B. K., Pluymert, K., Varjas, K., & Moore, R. (2002). *Exemplary mental health programs: School psychologists as mental health service providers* (3rd ed.). Silver Spring, MD: National Association of School Psychologists.

Nastasi, B. K., Schensul, J. J., deSilva, M. W. A., Varjas, K., Silva, K. T., Ratnayake, P., & Schensul, S. L. (1998–1999). Community-based sexual risk prevention program for Sri Lankan youth: Influencing sexual-risk decision making. *International Quarterly of Community Health Education, 18*(1), 139–155.

Nastasi, B. K., Schensul, J. J., Ratnayake, P., & Varjas, K. (1996). *Youth and sexual risk in Sri Lanka: Small group intervention. Program manual and facilitator guide*. Peradeniya, Sri Lanka: Centre for Intersectoral Community Health Studies.

Nastasi, B. K., Schensul, J. J., Tyler, C., Coe, C., Cintron, F., Araujo, R., et al. (2001). *The New Haven social development program social problem solving-cooperative education Grade 7 curriculum: Units I–III*. Hartford, CT: Institute for Community Research.

Nastasi, B. K., Varjas, K., Bernstein, R., Hellendoorn, C., Brewster, M., Hitchcock, J., et al. (1999). *Program for mental health promotion in Sri Lankan schools: Curriculum manual and instructional guide*. Albany: University at Albany, State University of New York, School Psychology Program.

Nastasi, B. K., Varjas, K., Bernstein, R., & Jayasena, A. (2000). Conducting participatory culture-specific consultation: A global perspective on multicultural consultation. *School Psychology Review, 29*, 401–413.

Nastasi, B. K., Varjas, K., Bernstein, R., & Pluymert, K. (1998a). *Exemplary mental health programs: School psychologists as mental health service providers* (2nd ed.). Silver Spring, MD: National Association of School Psychologists.

Nastasi, B. K., Varjas, K., Bernstein, R., & Pluymert, K. (1998b). Mental health programming and the role of school psychologists. *School Psychology Review, 27*, 217–232.

Nastasi, B. K., Varjas, K., Sarkar, S., & Jayasena, A. (1998). Participatory model of mental health programming: Lessons learned from work in a developing country. *School Psychology Review, 27*, 260–276.

Nastasi, B. K., Varjas, K., Schensul, S. L., Silva, K. T., Schensul, J. J., & Ratnayake, P. (2000). The participatory intervention model: A framework for conceptualizing and promoting intervention acceptability. *School Psychology Quarterly, 15*, 207–232.

National Advisory Mental Health Council. (1990). *National plan for research on child and adolescent mental disorders*. Washington, DC: National Institute of Mental Health.

National Association of School Psychologists. (1997). *School psychologists as health-care providers: Training packet*. Bethesda, MD: Author.

National Institute of Mental Health. (1990). *Research on children and adolescents with mental, behavioral, and developmental disorders* (DHHS Publications No. ADM-90-1659). Washington, DC: U.S. Government Printing Office.

National Institute of Mental Health. (1999, November 8). *Brief notes on the mental health of children and adolescents*. Retrieved June 29, 2001, from http://www.nimh.nih.gov/publicat/childnotes.cfm

National Institute of Mental Health. (2000). *Translating behavioral science into action: Report of the National Advisory Mental Health Council's Behavioral Science Workgroup* (NIMH Publication No. 00-4699). Washington, DC: U.S. Government Printing Office.

National Institute of Mental Health. (2001a). *Blueprint for change: Research on child and adolescent mental health: Report of the National Advisory Mental Health Council Workgroup on Child and Adolescent Mental Health Intervention Development and Deployment*. Washington, DC: Author.

National Institute of Mental Health. (2001b, January). *Women hold up half the sky: Women and mental health research* (NIMH Publication No. 01-4607). Retrieved March 8, 2003, from http://www.nimh.nih.gov/publicat/womensoms.cfm#20

National Resource Network for Child and Family Mental Health Services at the Washington Business Group on Health. (Ed.). (1999). *A compilation of lessons learned from the 22 grantees of the 1997 Comprehensive Community Mental Health Services for Children and Their Families Program. In Systems of Care: Promising practices in children's mental health, 1998 Series* (Vol. VII). Washington, DC: Center for Effective Collaboration and Practice, American Institutes for Research.

Nelson, J. R., Dykman, C., Powell, S., & Petty, D. (1996). The effects of a group counseling intervention on students with behavioral adjustment problems. *Elementary School Guidance & Counseling, 31*(1), 21–33.

Nitz, K. (1999). Adolescent pregnancy prevention: A review of interventions and programs. *Clinical Psychology Review, 19*, 457–471.

Nixon, C. T., & Northrup, D. A. (Eds.). (1997). *Children's mental health services: Vol. 3. Evaluating mental health services: How do programs for children "work" in the real world?* Thousand Oaks, CA: Sage.

Noell, J., Ary, D., & Duncan, T. (1997). Development and evaluation of a sexual decision-making and social skills program: "The choice is yours—preventing HIV/STDs." *Health Education and Behavior, 24*(1), 87–101.

O'Dea, J. A., & Abraham, S. (2000). Improving the body image, eating attitudes, and behaviors of young male and female adolescents: A new educational approach that focused on self-esteem. *International Journal of Eating Disorders, 28*(1), 43–47.

Office of the Press Secretary. (2002, April 29). *President's New Freedom Commission on Mental Health: Executive order.* Washington, DC: White House. Retrieved August 29, 2002, from http://www.whitehouse.gov/news/releases/22020429-2.html

Osher, D., & Hanley, T. V. (1996). Implications of the National Agenda to Improve Results for Children and Youth With or At Risk of Serious Emotional Disturbance. In R. J. Illback & C. M. Nelson (Eds.), *Emerging school-based approaches for children with emotional or behavioral problems* (pp. 7–36). Hillsdale, NJ: Erlbaum.

Osofsky, J. D. (1995). The effects of exposure to violence on young children. *American Psychologist, 50,* 782–788.

Paavola, J. C., Carey, K., Cobb, C., Illback, R. J., Joseph, H. M. Jr., Routh, d. K., & Torruella, A. (1996). Interdisciplinary school practice: Implications of the service integration movement for psychologists. *Professional Psychology: Research and Practice, 27,* 34–40.

Patterson, J. M. (1996). Family research methods: Issues and strategies. In C. A. Heflinger & C. T. Nixon (Eds.), *Children's mental health services: Vol. 2. Families and the mental health system for children and adolescents* (pp. 117–144). Thousand Oaks, CA: Sage.

Pedro-Carroll, J. (1997). The Children of Divorce Intervention Program: Fostering resilient outcomes for school-aged children. In G. W. Albee & T. P. Gullotta (Eds.), *Primary prevention works: Vol. 6. Issues in children's and families' lives* (pp. 213–238). Thousand Oaks, CA: Sage.

Perry, C. L., & Kelder, S. H. (1992). Models for effective prevention. *Journal of Adolescent Health, 13,* 355–363.

Phillips, B. N. (1999). Strengthening the links between science and practice: Reading, evaluating, and applying research in school psychology. In C. R. Reynolds & T. B. Gutkin (Eds.), *Handbook of school psychology* (3rd ed., pp. 56–77). New York: Wiley.

Pitcher, G., & Poland, S. (1992). *Crisis intervention in the schools.* New York: Guilford Press.

Policy Leadership Cadre for Mental Health in Schools. (2001, May). *Mental health in schools: Guidelines, models, resources, and policy considerations.* Los Angeles: University of California, Department of Psychology, Center for Mental Health in Schools. Retrieved from http://smhp.psych.ucla.edu

Poulin, F., & Dishion, T. J. (1997, April). *Iatrogenic effects among high risk adolescents aggregated within interventions: An analysis of the durability and process.* Paper presented at the Society for Research in Child Development, Washington, DC.

Power, T. J. (2000). Commentary. The school psychologist as community-focused, public health professional: Emerging challenges and implications for training. *School Psychology Review, 29,* 557–559.

Power, T. J., DuPaul, G. J., Shapiro, E. S., & Parrish, J. M. (1995). Pediatric school psychology: The emergence of a subspecialty. *School Psychology Review, 24,* 244–257.

Power, T. J., Manz, P. H., & Leff, S. S. (2003). Training for effective practice in schools. In M. D. Weist, S. W. Evans, & N. A. Lever (Eds.), *Handbook of school mental health* (pp. 257–274). New York: Kluwer Academic.

Prout, S. M., & Prout, H. T. (1998). A meta-analysis of school-based studies of counseling and psychotherapy: An update. *Journal of School Psychology, 36,* 121–136.

Reschly, D. J. (2000). The present and future status of school psychology in the United States. *School Psychology Review, 29,* 507–522.

Reschly, D. J., & Wilson, M. S. (1995). School psychology practitioners and faculty: 1986 to 1991–92 trends in demographics, roles, satisfaction, and system reform. *School Psychology Review, 24,* 62–80.

Reynolds, C. R., & Kamphaus, R. W. (1992). *Behavior Assessment System for Children (BASC) manual.* Circle Pines, MN: American Guidance Service.

Reynolds, W. R. (1986). A model for the screening and identification of depressed children and adolescents in school settings. *Professional School Psychology, 1,* 117–130.

Ring-Kurtz, S. E., Sonnichsen, S., & Hoover-Dempsey, K. V. (1995). School-based mental health services for children. In L. Bickman & D. J. Rog (Eds.), *Children's mental health services: Vol. 1. Research, policy, and evaluation* (pp. 117–144). Thousand Oaks, CA: Sage.

Roberts, M. C. (Ed.). (1996). *Model programs in child and family mental health.* Mahwah, NJ: Erlbaum.

Roberts, M. C., Carlson, C. I., Erickson, M. T., Friedman, R. M., La Greca, A. M., Lemanek, K. L., et al. (1998). A model for training psychologists to provide services for children and adolescents. *Professional Psychology: Research and Practice, 29,* 293–299.

Roberts, M. C., & Hinton-Nelson, M. (1996). Models for service delivery in child and family mental health. In M. C. Roberts (Ed.), *Model programs in child and family mental health* (pp. 1–22). Mahwah, NJ: Erlbaum.

Robinson, W. L., Ruch-Ross, H. S., Watkins-Ferrell, P., & Lightfoot, S. (1993). Risk behavior in adolescence: Methodological challenges in school-based research. *School Psychology Quarterly, 8,* 241–254.

Rones, M., & Hoagwood, K. (2000). School-based mental health services: A research review. *Clinical Child and Family Psychology Review, 3,* 223–241.

Rosenfield, S. A., & Gravois, T. A. (1996). *Instructional consultation teams: Collaborating for change.* New York: Guilford Press.

Ryan, G. W., & Bernard, H. R. (2000). Data management and analysis methods. In N. K. Denzin & Y. S. Lincoln (Eds.), *Handbook of qualitative research* (2nd ed., pp. 769–801). Thousand Oaks, CA: Sage.

Sandoval, J., & Brock, S. E. (1996). The school psychologist's role in suicide prevention. *School Psychology Quarterly, 11,* 169–185.

Saxe, L., Cross, T. P., Lovas, G. S., & Gardner, J. K. (1995). Evaluation of the mental health services for youth: Examining rhetoric in action. In L. Bickman & D. J. Rog (Eds.), *Children's mental health services: Vol. 1. Research, policy, and evaluation* (pp. 206–235). Thousand Oaks, CA: Sage.

Schensul, J. J. (1998). Community-based risk prevention with urban youth. *School Psychology Review, 27,* 233–245.

Schensul, J. J. (1998–1999). Learning about sexual meaning and decision-making from urban adolescents. *International Quarterly of Community Health Education, 18*(1), 29–48.

Schensul, J. J. (2001). [Pathways to drug use]. Unpublished raw data. Hartford, CT: Institute for Community Research.

Schensul, J. J., & LeCompte, M. D. (Eds.). (1999). *Ethnographer's toolkit* (Vols. 1–7). Walnut Creek, CA: AltaMira.

Schensul, J. J., & Schensul, S. L. (1992). Collaborative research: Methods of inquiry for social change. In M. D. LeCompte, W. L. Millroy, & J. Preissle (Eds.), *The handbook of qualitative research in education* (pp. 161–200). San Diego, CA: Academic Press.

Schensul, S. L., Schensul, J. J., & LeCompte, M. D. (1999). *Essential ethnographic methods: Observations, interviews, and questionnaires—Ethnographer's toolkit, Book 2.* Walnut Creek, CA: AltaMira.

Schinke, S. P. (1998). Preventing teenage pregnancy: Translating research knowledge. *Journal of Human Behavior in the Social Environment, 1*(1), 53–66.

Schoenwald, S. K., Henggeler, S. W., Pickrel, S. G., & Cunningham, P. B. (1996). Treating seriously troubled youths and families in their contexts: Multisystemic therapy. In M. C. Roberts (Ed.), *Model programs in child and family mental health* (pp. 317–332). Mahwah, NJ: Erlbaum.

Schorr, L. B. (1997). *Common purpose: Strengthening families and neighborhoods to rebuild America.* New York: Anchor.

Schwab-Stone, M., Ayers, T., Kasprow, W., Voyce, C., Barone, C., Shriver, T., & Weissberg, R. (1995). No safe haven: A study of violence exposure in an urban community. *Journal of the American Academy of Child and Adolescent Psychiatry, 34,* 1343–1352.

Segall, M. H., Lonner, W. J., & Berry, J. W. (1998). Cross-cultural psychology as a scholarly discipline: On the flowering of culture in behavioral research. *American Psychologist, 53,* 1101–1110.

Sells, C. W., & Blum, W. R. (1996). Current trends in adolescent health. In R. J. DiClemente, W. B. Hansen, & L. E. Ponton (Eds.), *Handbook of adolescent health risk behavior* (pp. 5–34). New York: Plenum.

Serrano-Garcia, I. (1990). Implementing research: Putting our values to work. In P. Tolan, C. Keys, F. Chertok, & L. Jason (Eds.), *Researching community psychology: Issues of theory and methods* (pp. 171–182). Washington, DC: American Psychological Association.

Shapiro, E. S., & DuPaul, G. J. (1996). A school-based consultation program for service delivery to middle school students with attention-deficit/hyperactivity disorder. *Journal of Emotional and Behavioral Disorders, 4*(2), 73–81.

Shapiro, E. S., & Elliott, S. N. (1999). Curriculum-based assessment and other performance-based assessment strategies. In C. R. Reynolds & T. B. Gutkin (Eds.), *Handbook of school psychology* (3rd ed., pp. 383–408). New York: Wiley.

Sheley, J. R., & Wright, J. D. (1995). *In the line of fire: Youth, guns, and violence in urban America.* New York: Aldine De Gruyter.

Sheridan, S. M., Dee, C. C., Morgan, J. C., McCormick, M. E., & Walker, D. (1996). A multimethod intervention for social skills deficits in children with ADHD and their parents. *School Psychology Review, 25*, 57–76.

Sheridan, S. M., & Gutkin, T. B. (2000). The ecology of school psychology: Examining and changing our paradigm for the 21st century. *School Psychology Review, 29*, 485–502.

Sheridan, S. M., Kratochwill, T. R., & Bergan, J. R. (1996). *Conjoint behavioral consultation.* New York: Plenum.

Sheridan, S. M., & Walker, D. (1999). Social skills in context: Considerations for assessment, intervention, and generalization. In C. R. Reynolds & T. B. Gutkin (Eds.), *Handbook of school psychology* (3rd ed., pp. 686–708). New York: Wiley.

Short, R. J., & Rosenthal, S. L. (1995). Expanding roles or evolving identity? Doctoral school psychologists in school vs. nonschool settings. *Psychology in the Schools, 32*, 296–305.

Shure, M. B. (1996). I Can Problem Solve (ICPS): An interpersonal cognitive problem solving program for children. In M. C. Roberts (Ed.), *Model programs in child and family mental health* (pp. 47–62). Mahwah, NJ: Erlbaum.

Silva, K. T., Schensul, S. L., Schensul, J. J., Nastasi, B. K., de Silva, M. W. A., Sivayoganathan, C., et al. (1997). *Women and AIDS Research Program: Youth and sexual risk in Sri Lanka.* Washington, DC: International Center for Research on Women.

Smith, C. A. (1997). Factors associated with early sexual activity among urban adolescents. *Social Work, 42*, 334–344.

Smith, M. U., & DiClemente, R. J. (2000). STAND: A peer educator training curriculum for sexual reduction in the rural south. *Preventive Medicine, 30*, 441–449.

Smith, S., & Coutinho, M. J. (1997). Achieving the goals of the national agenda: Progress and prospects. *Journal of Emotional and Behavioral Disorders, 5*, 2–5.

Sourander, A., Helstela, L., Helenius, H., & Piha, J. (2000). Persistence of bullying from childhood to adolescence: A longitudinal 8-year follow-up study. *Child Abuse and Neglect, 24,* 873–881.

Spradley, J. P. (1979). *The ethnographic interview.* New York: Holt, Rinehart & Winston.

Spradley, J. P. (1980). *Participant observation.* New York: Holt, Rinehart & Winston.

Stark, K. D., Brookman, C. S., & Frazier, R. (1990). A comprehensive school-based treatment program for depressed children. *School Psychology Quarterly, 5,* 111–140.

Steiner, G. L. (1990). Children, families, and AIDS: Psychosocial and psychotherapeutic aspects. *New Jersey Psychologist, 40,* 11–14.

Stoiber, K. C., & Kratochwill, T. R. (2000). Empirically supported interventions and school psychology: Part I. Rationale and methodological issues. *School Psychology Quarterly, 15,* 75–105.

Stokols, D. (1992). Establishing and maintaining health environments: Toward a social ecology of health promotion. *American Psychologist, 47,* 6–22.

Stoner, G., & Green, S. K. (1992). Reconsidering the scientist–practitioner model for school psychology practice. *School Psychology Review, 21,* 155–166.

Strauss, A., & Corbin, J. (1990). *Basics of qualitative research: Grounded theory procedures and techniques.* Thousand Oaks, CA: Sage.

Talley, R. C., & Short, R. J. (1996). Social reforms and the future of school practice: Implications for American psychology. *Professional Psychology: Research and Practice, 27,* 5–13.

Taylor, L., & Adelman, H. S. (2000). Toward ending the marginalization and fragmentation of mental health in schools. *Journal of School Health, 70,* 210–215.

Tremblay, R. E., Pagani-Kurtz, L., Masse, L. C., Vitaro, F., & Pihl, R. O. (1995). A bimodal preventive intervention for disruptive kindergarten boys: Its impact through mid-adolescence. *Journal of Consulting and Clinical Psychology, 63,* 560–568.

U.S. Department of Education. (2002a). *A new era: Revitalizing special education for children and their families.* Washington, DC: U.S. Department of Education, Office of Special Education and Rehabilitative Services.

U.S. Department of Education. (2002b). *No Child Left Behind: A desktop reference.* Washington, DC: U.S. Department of Education, Office of Elementary and Secondary Education.

U.S. Department of Health and Human Services. (1993). *Child health USA '93* (DHHS Publication No. HRSA-MCH-94-1). Washington, DC: U.S. Government Printing Office.

U.S. Department of Health and Human Services. (1999). *Mental health: A report of the Surgeon General.* Rockville, MD: U.S. Department of Health and Human Services, Office of the Surgeon General, Substance Abuse and Mental Health Services Administration.

U.S. Department of Health and Human Services. (2001a). *Mental health: Culture, race, and ethnicity—A supplement to mental health: A report of the Surgeon General.* Rockville, MD: U.S. Department of Health and Human Services, Office of the Surgeon General, Substance Abuse and Mental Health Services Administration.

U.S. Department of Health and Human Services. (2001b). *Youth violence: A report of the Surgeon General.* Rockville, MD: U.S. Department of Health and Human Services, Office of the Surgeon General, Substance Abuse and Mental Health Services Administration.

U.S. Secret Service and U.S. Department of Education. (2002). *Threat assessment in schools: A guide to managing threatening situations and to creating safe school climates.* Washington, DC: Author.

Varjas, K. M. (2003). *A participatory culture-specific consultation (PCSC) approach to intervention development.* Unpublished doctoral dissertation, University at Albany, State University of New York.

Vossekuil, B., Fein, R. A., Reddy, M., Borum, R., & Modzeleski, W. (2002, May). *The final report and findings of the Safe School Initiative: Implications for the prevention of school attacks in the United States.* Washington, DC: U.S. Secret Service and U.S. Department of Education.

Walter, H. J., Vaughan, R. D., Armstrong, B., Krakoff, R. Y., Tiezzi, L., & McCarthy, J. F. (1995). School-based health care for urban minority junior high school students. *Archives of Pediatric and Adolescent Medicine, 149,* 1221–1225.

Wang, M. C., Haertel, G. D., & Walberg, H. J. (1998). Effective features of collaborative, school-linked services for children in elementary schools: What do we know from research and practice? *LSS Publication Series No. 98* (2), 1–14. Retrieved October 15, 1999, from http://www.temple.edu/LSS/pub98-2.htm

Weissberg, R. P. (1990). Fidelity and adaptation: Combining the best of both perspectives. In P. Tolan, C. Keys, F. Chertok, & L. Jason (Eds.), *Researching community psychology: Issues of theory and methods* (pp. 186–189). Washington, DC: American Psychological Association.

Weissberg, R. P., Caplan, M., & Harwood, R. L. (1991). Promoting competent young people in competence-enhancing environments: A systems-based perspective on primary prevention. *Journal of Consulting and Clinical Psychology, 59,* 830–841.

Weissberg, R. P., & Elias, M. J. (1993). Enhancing young people's social competence and health behavior: An important challenge for educators, scientists, policymakers, and funders. *Applied and Preventive Psychology, 2,* 179–190.

Weist, M. D., Myers, C. P., Hastings, E. H., Ghuman, H., & Han, Y. L. (1999). Psychosocial functioning of youth receiving mental health services in the schools versus community mental health centers. *Community Mental Health Journal, 35*(1), 69–81.

Weist, M. D., Paskewitz, D. A., Warner, B. S., & Flaherty, L. T. (1996). Treatment outcome of school-based mental health services for urban teenagers. *Community Mental Health Journal, 32,* 149–157.

Weisz, J. R., Donenberg, G. R., Han, S. S., & Kauneckis, D. (1995). Child and adolescent psychotherapy outcomes in experiments versus clinics: Why the disparity? *Journal of Abnormal Child Psychology*, 83–106.

Werthamer-Larsson, L. (1994). Methodological issues in school-based services research. *Journal of Clinical Child Psychology*, *23*, 121–132.

Wickstrom, K. F., Jones, K. M., LaFleur, L. H., & Witt, J. C. (1998). An analysis of treatment integrity in school-based behavioral consultation. *School Psychology Quarterly*, *13*, 141–154.

Wolcott, H. F. (1994). *Transforming qualitative data: Description, analysis, and interpretation*. Thousand Oaks, CA: Sage.

Ysseldyke, J. E., & Christenson, S. L. (2002). *FAAB: Functional assessment of academic behavior: Creating successful learning environments*. Longmont, CO: Sopris West.

Ysseldyke, J. E., & Elliott, J. (1999). Effective instructional practices: Implications for assessing instructional environments. In C. R. Reynolds & T. B. Gutkin (Eds.), *Handbook of school psychology* (3rd ed., pp. 497–518). New York: Wiley.

Zill, N., & Schoenborn, C. A. (1990, November 16). *Developmental, learning, and emotional problems: Health of our nation's children, United States, 1988* (Advanced data from National Center for Health Statistics, No. 190). Hyattsville, MD: Public Health Service.

AUTHOR INDEX

Vitaro, F., 117
Vossekuil, B., 10

Walberg, H. J., 20n.2, 23
Walker, D., 41, 118, 123
Walker, K. J., 25
Walter, H. J., 21, 29
Wang, M. C., 20n.2, 23, 29, 30
Warner, B. S., 118
Watkins-Ferrell, P., 138
Watson, M., 114
Weed, S., 29
Weissberg, R. P., 21, 22, 38, 67n.4
Weist, M. D., 23, 29, 30, 118, 138
Weisz, J. R., 20n.2
Wells, A. M., 20n.2, 30
Werthamer-Larsson, L., 138

West, S. G., 138
Whitehouse, S., 22
Whitman, T. L., 132
Whyte, W. F., 35
Wickstrom, K. F., 37
Williams, S., 152, 156
Wilson, M. S., 25
Windle, M., 138
Witt, J. C., 30, 37, 132
Wolcott, H. F., 42n.2, 48
Wright, J. D., 10

Ysseldyke, J. E., 41

Zill, N., 6
Zins, J. E., 38

SUBJECT INDEX

Involvement, *continued*
    of school psychologists in compre-
        hensive mental health services,
        26
    of stakeholders, 132–133

Jayasena, Asoka, 62
Journals, 50, 51, 148–149
Juvenile offenders, 9, 10

Learning, social morbidities and decrease
    in, 6
Learning the culture (phase 2), 61,
    85–89
    analyses of data in, 87
    data collection guidelines for, 85, 87
    focus of, 85
    goal of, 61
    key considerations for, 86
    sample interview questions for,
        87–89
    in SLMH Project, 61, 73
Leff, Stephen, 125
Life Skills Training (LST), 114
Lifestyle, 7
Local theory. *See* Culture-specific theory
    or model (phase 6)
Logs, 148–149
LST *(Life Skills Training)*, 114

Male Sexual Health Concerns and
    Prevention of HIV/STDs project,
    132n.3
Manic-depressive illness, 7
Marijuana, 12, 13
MDMA, 13
Member checks, 50, 51
Mental health
    definition of, 4, 5
    as national and global priority, 6
    promotion of, 111
    as public health, 4, 5
Mental health problems, xiii
    in children and adolescents, 5–7
    definition of, 4, 5
    and exposure to violence, 10
    far-reaching effects of, 6

Mental health services
    access to, 19
    school psychologists engaged in,
        25–27
    U.S. Surgeon General's recommenda-
        tions on, 42n.3
Mental illness or disorders. *See also*
        Psychiatric disorders
    adults with, 6
    childhood disability/morbidity/mor-
        tality caused by, xiii
    definition of, 4, 5
Methamphetamine, 12
Methods
    for capacity building phase, 158
    for culture-specific theory/model
        phase, 105
    ethnographic, 85, 143–151
    for existing theory/research/practice
        phase, 81
    for formative research phase, 96, 98
    for forming partnerships phase, 90
    for goal/problem identification
        phase, 95
    for learning the culture phase, 86
    of naturalistic inquiry, 43
    for program design phase, 113
    for program evaluation phase, 134,
        138–143
    for program implementation phase,
        128
    for translation phase, 160
Minority groups, 18–19
Models, xiii. *See also* Participatory
        culture-specific intervention
        model
    collaborative (participatory), 37–38
    for continuum of service, 111,
        114–118
    ecological, 5
    for multiple perspectives assessment,
        136
    public health model, 4, 5
    traditional vs. PCSIM, 33–35
Modifications. *See* Adaptation(s)
Motor vehicle accidents
    and alcohol use, 13
    deaths from, 7, 8
Multiple perspectives model, 136
Multisite projects, program
        implementation/evaluation in, 22

NASP (National Association of School Psychologists), 25

Nastasi, B. K., 62

National Association of School Psychologists (NASP), 25

National Association of School Psychologists Survey of Mental Health Programs, 164–171

National Institute of Mental Health, 6–7, 18n.1, 181

National Institute of Mental Health Workgroup on Child and Adolescent Mental Health Intervention Development and Deployment, 71

Natural adaptation, 67, 126. *See also* Program implementation (phase 8)

Naturalistic inquiry, 42–43. *See also* Ethnography

Negative case analysis, 50, 51

Neglect, 9

Negotiation
    of educational priorities, 183
    and participatory consultation, 37
    of partnerships, 58, 61
    skills in, 89
    of stakeholders' perspectives, 66

Networks, 151

Observation, 50, 51, 145, 147–148

Opportunities
    in capacity building phase, 159
    in culture-specific theory/model phase, 106
    in existing theory/research/practice phase, 82
    in formative research phase, 97
    in forming partnerships phase, 90
    in goal/problem identification phase, 95
    in learning the culture phase, 86
    in program design phase, 113
    in program evaluation phase, 135
    in program implementation phase, 128
    in translation phase, 161

Outcomes, evaluation of, 141

Ownership (by stakeholders), 132–133

Oxfam, 152

PAR. *See* Participatory action research

Parent–school early intervention programs, 117

Participants
    in capacity building phase, 158
    in culture-specific theory/model phase, 105
    in existing theory/research/practice phase, 81
    in formative research phase, 96
    in forming partnerships phase, 90
    in goal/problem identification phase, 95
    in learning the culture phase, 86
    in program design phase, 112
    in program evaluation phase, 134
    in program implementation phase, 127
    in translation phase, 160

Participation, collaboration vs., 37n.1

Participatory action research (PAR), 35–37

Participatory consultation, 37–39, 131

Participatory consultation model, 89

Participatory culture-specific consultation, 38, 39

Participatory culture-specific intervention model (PCSIM), xiii–xiv, 33–52. *See also specific phases*
    broader application of, xiv
    capacity building phase of, 69–70
    challenges in applying, 183–186
    culture-specific theory or model phase of, 64, 65
    ecological perspective in, 38–41
    ethnography in, 42–51
    existing theory, research, and practice phase of, 59–61
    formative (research) components of, 59–65
    formative research phase of, 63–64
    forming partnerships phase of, 61–62
    foundational components of, 35
    goal or problem identification phase of, 63
    as integration of research and intervention, 53–55
    learning the culture phase of, 61
    main components of, 54, 56–58

Risks
   comprehensive programs for reducing, 21
   and intervention activity, 176–177
   for posttraumatic stress syndrome, 11

Satcher, David, 3
Saxe, L., 22
Schizophrenia, 7
School-based mental health services, xiii, xiv, 24–27, 118. *See also* Comprehensive school-based mental health programs
School difficulties
   and exposure to stressors, 11
   and poverty, 17
School psychologists
   as advocates, 3
   changing role/identity of, 185–186
   as mental health care providers, 26–27
   as reflective practitioners, 36–37
   reported uses of time by, 25–26
   school-based mental health services role of, 24–27
   traditional roles of, 24
School psychology
   ecological perspective in, 40–41
   future directions for, 186–189
Schools
   demand for increased participation by, 24
   drugs acquired in, 13
   and Level IV treatment services, 118
   mental health care received through, 19
   need for mental health services in, 5–6
   violence in, 8–10
   weapons in, 9–10
School shootings, 10, 119
Science based interventions, 56n.1
Scientifically based interventions, 56n.1
Screening
   for early intervention, 117
   for risk reduction, 115–116
SDP (Social Development Program), 125
Secondary-level students, most prevalent disorders in, 6
Segmentation (of phases), 94

Self-evaluation skills, 93
Service coordination and integration, 118–123
   cautions in, 120–121
   illustration of, 119, 121–123
   insights and recommendations in, 120
Sexual abuse, 9
Sexual activity, 14–17
Sexually-transmitted diseases (STDs), 14, 15
Sexual risk prevention programs, 14, 150
Skills
   for capacity building phase, 158
   for culture-specific theory/model phase, 105
   for existing theory/research/practice phase, 81
   for formative research phase, 96
   for forming partnerships phase, 86, 90, 92, 93
   for goal/problem identification phase, 95
   for learning the culture phase, 86
   for parents and community members, 124
   for program design phase, 113
   for program evaluation phase, 135
   for program implementation phase, 128
   for translation phase, 160
SLMH. *See* Sri Lanka Mental Health Project
Social–cultural factors, PTSD risk and, 11
Social Development Program (SDP), 125
Social morbidity(-ies), xiii, 7–19
   deaths caused by, 7–8
   definition of, 7
   dietary behaviors as, 17–18
   drug use and abuse as, 11–13
   educational results of, 6
   poverty as, 17
   sexual activity as, 14–17
   suicide as, 8
   violence as, 8–11
Social networks, 151, 178–179
Social rejection, HIV/AIDS and, 16
Social validity, 68, 140, 142
Socio–cultural variations, services addressing, 30

Socioeconomic conditions
    and HIV/AIDS, 16
    psychological/social problems related
        to, 17
Spatial mapping, 102–103
Special education students
    assessment for eligibility as, 25
    suicide by, 8
Sri Lanka Mental Health Project
        (SLMH), 57–71, 73–78
    application of PCSIM to, 57
    capacity building phase in, 70, 77
    culture-specific theory or model
        phase in, 64, 65, 75, 106–107
    ethnographic surveys in, 143–145
    existing theory, research, and prac-
        tice phase in, 59–61, 73, 82–83
    focused group interviews in,
        100–102
    formative research phase in, 63–64,
        74
    forming partnerships phase in, 62,
        74
    goal or problem identification phase
        in, 63, 74
    learning the culture phase in, 61, 73
    partners in, 58–59
    program design phase in, 66–67, 76
    program evaluation phase in, 69, 76
    program implementation phase in,
        68, 76
    risk reduction in, 115
    translation phase in, 71, 78
Staff development, 131–132
Stakeholders
    acceptability of comprehensive pro-
        grams to, 21
    active participation of, 53, 54
    communities as, 124
    definition of, 79n.1
    establishing relationships among, 61
    families as, 124
    goal identification by, 63
    in group decision making, 94
    identifying personal theories of, 84
    independent functioning of, 70
    involvement/ownership/
        empowerment of, 132–133
    negotiating multiple perspectives of,
        66
    as partners, 89

process of engaging, 37, 38
program planner interactions with,
    82
responsibility of, 58
in school-based mental health pro-
    grams, 58
in translation phase, 161
STAND (Stand Together Against Negative
        Decisions), 114
STDs. See Sexually-transmitted diseases
Steroids, 12
Stigma (associated with mental illness),
    19
Strategies
    for capacity building phase, 158
    for culture-specific theory/model
        phase, 105
    for existing theory/research/practice
        phase, 81, 83–84
    for formative research phase, 96
    for forming partnerships phase, 90
    for goal/problem identification
        phase, 95
    for learning the culture phase, 86
    for program design phase, 113
    for program evaluation phase, 134
    for program implementation phase,
        128
    for translation phase, 160
Stressors, exposure to, 11
Substance abuse, 11–13
    in adults with mental disorders, 6
    and bullying, 11
    and eating disorders, 17
Substance Abuse and Mental Health Ser-
        vices Administration, 18n.1
Suicidal behavior, 6, 8, 11
Suicide, 7, 8
"Supported by outcomes research," 56n.1
Surveys, ethnographic, 143–145
Sustainability, 141, 142. See also Capacity
        building (phase 10)
Systems of care, 118

Tasks
    in capacity building phase, 158
    in culture-specific theory/model
        phase, 105
    in existing theory/research/practice
        phase, 81

ABOUT THE AUTHORS

Bonnie Kaul Nastasi received her PhD from Kent State University in 1986. She is associate director of interventions at the Institute for Community Research, a nonprofit research organization in Hartford, Connecticut, and former program director and associate professor of school psychology at the University at Albany, State University of New York. She has conducted applied research and has published books, chapters, and journal articles on mental health and health risk among school-age and young adult populations in the United States and internationally, particularly in South Asia. Her interests include mental health promotion, health risk prevention, use of qualitative research methods in psychology, and promoting school psychology internationally. She is currently an associate editor of *School Psychology Review* and has served on the editorial boards of a number of psychology and education journals.

Rachel Bernstein Moore completed her PsyD in school psychology at the University at Albany, State University of New York. She is currently working as a school psychologist in the Schenectady city school district in New York. Her research interests include school-based mental health promotion and the role of school psychologists in mental health programming. She has numerous publications and presentations on the topic of school-based mental health promotion for children and adolescents.

Kristen M. Varjas received her PsyD in school psychology from the University at Albany, State University of New York. She is currently an assistant professor in the Counseling and Psychological Services Department at Georgia State University, Atlanta. She has conducted applied research on mental health and health risk among school-age and adult populations in the United

States and Sri Lanka. Her interests include international and national mental health promotion, developing culture-specific prevention and intervention programs, and developing culturally appropriate school psychology practice. She recently received awards from the Georgia Association of School Psychologists and Georgia State University for her work with diverse populations in the United States and Sri Lanka.